PROGNOSTICATION

Principles and Practice

Bernardo Gutierrez, MD

PAGE PUBLISHING
Conneaut Lake, PA

First originally published by Page Publishing 2024

ISBN 979-8-88960-938-4 (pbk)
ISBN 979-8-88960-960-5 (digital)

Printed in the United States of America

I dedicate this book to my wife for her unconditional love
and support throughout my long career, never faltering
and always believing in me. Also, to my children who have
supported and helped me in the last steps of the process.

CONTENTS

CHAPTER 1
Overview of Prognostication

The practice of medicine has become scientifically complex. While aggressive and potentially lifesaving therapies have emerged for even the deadliest of diseases, physicians need to recognize that many of these advanced treatments are not appropriate for all patients. This is particularly true for the elderly. Many elderly patients do not have the physical reserves that they would need to recover functionality and thus may not be able to tolerate even the temporary negative effects of aggressive care. To combat this problem, physicians need to gain expertise in the art and process of prognostication, which is a method or process that can be used to predict future outcomes based on a critical evaluation of current knowledge. The process of prognostication needs not be complex or time-consuming. At its core, prognostication uses standard clinical observations to help physicians predict the relative benefits of aggressive and potentially curative *versus* supportive and typically more palliative care for each patient case. In this chapter, we review the basic issues involved in identifying appropriate medical care for elderly patients and provide a general overview of how prognostication can assist in this process in routine clinical practice.

Objectives

The goals of this section are as follows:

- To understand the problem
- To recognize the importance of prognostication with respect to the practice of medicine in a changing population

- To provide a general overview of the theory and practice of prognostication
- To appreciate the physician's perspective on prognostication
- To identify the advantages of prognostication in the practice of medicine

Introduction

The practice of medicine is currently in the midst of crisis in the United States (US). While our country expends the highest percentage of the gross national product on health care of any nation in the developed world, the US scores among the lowest on metrics that evaluate the quality of health care provided to its residents. The health care system is not providing people with what they need. Many complex factors contribute to this problem.

Perhaps first and foremost, medicine in the US evolved based on a purely scientific model. This approach undoubtedly led to many significant advances in medical science. The US is certainly one of the countries with superior medical knowledge. At current writing, there are medical specialists that focus on almost every type of condition or disease. With this increase in knowledge, the expectations of the general public have also increased, and the common understanding is that specific diseases need to be treated by dedicated specialists.

While this specialized approach has worked and continues to work well for patients with single medical issues, it tends to complicate the care of those with complex multisystem conditions. This is particularly evident in the care of hospitalized patients who are typically referred to different physicians for their numerous problems. In these cases, the oversight provided by the primary care physician frequently becomes diluted, and the patients lose critical continuity of care. Currently specialist-based care typically focuses on a single disease process and uses established protocols with little to no consideration of whether a given treatment is appropriate for a particular patient. Patients with more than one disease or disorder are frequently asked to see many physicians, often a single specialist for each medical issue. In these cases, no one claims sole responsibility for the patient's medical care. While this approach has worked reasonably well for patients with single issues, it certainly does not address the medical concerns of the overall population.

The characteristics of the patient population in the US are currently changing.[1] Not only is the population increasing in size, but the inhabitants are also generally older, weaker, and more dependent on medical care; these individuals frequently present with many highly complex medical issues. Thus far, no evidence-based standards of care have been developed to manage patients with multisystem disorders.[2] Furthermore, variabilities associated with different rates of aging are significant enough to require reconsideration of many of the current methods used for medical standardization. Enforcing these outdated standards will create unwanted, unnecessarily expensive, and futile medical care. It is also critical to recognize that we are just at the beginning of this period of massive change. The most significant changes in population dynamics have just begun, and they are predicted to continue for the next several decades.

Many individuals in our society have developed unrealistic expectations of modern medicine and believe that physicians can cure all diseases and thus prolong life. Many individuals perceive death as a punishable failure on the part of the physician. The liability concerns that have developed based on this unreasonable perception together with the commercialization of medicine, the introduction of the concept of productivity in medical practice, and the current economic crisis have all challenged the practice of medicine and have placed physicians at a critical crossroads.

As a final point, it is also important to understand that the current system profits by keeping the patient sick and in need of more (and more expensive) care. This system is unlikely to change, especially because many of the stakeholders (notably those in the medical insurance industry) are more or less happy with the way things are right now.

---

[1] *National Vital Statistics Report* 71, no. 1 (2022).

[2] I. Ratnani, S. Fatima, M. Abid, Z. Surani, S. Surani, "Evidence-Based Medicine: History, Review, Criticisms, and Pitfalls," *Cureus* 15, no. 2 (2023), e35266.

All these factors working together have created a health care system based on profit-making, rather than on the medical needs of the patients.

This system needs to change soon. The challenge to evoking change is, by its nature, complex, and in this case, there is no simple or straightforward solution. However, one thing that physicians can do in the meantime is to change the way they approach the care of the individual patient. In a large sense, the practice of medicine needs to go back to basics. Physicians need to begin by evaluating their complex patients individually and personalizing their care based on their unique situations.[3] In short, physicians need to make the best out of each encounter with every patient in their practice.

Of course, not all changes are bad. Computer-based systematization of patient information has been good overall for the practice of medicine. Today physicians in almost every setting will have access to all the pertinent information needed to make the appropriate decisions for nearly every patient. However, physicians still need to learn to identify and analyze crucial information and to understand its significance in determining the future of a given patient. This process is known as *prognostication*.

Prognostication is a process that will permit the physician to evaluate individual patients and the extent of their declining health by judging their strength (*i.e.*, normal to poor, secondary to aging or disease). Based on this information, the physician will then be able to determine if a recommended clinical protocol will or will not be of benefit to the patient.

What is prognostication? According to the dictionary, a *prognosis* is "a forecast or prediction of the probable course and/or outcome of a disease." Thus, *prognostication* is a method used to process information. When introduced as part of the regular practice of medicine, this method can be used to determine possible outcomes for a given patient. This practice has evolved over time.

---

[3] S. Mathur, J. Sutton, "Personalized Medicine Could Transform Healthcare," *Biomed Reps* 7 (2017): 3–5.

In the past, clinicians were frequently tasked with determining when and if there was nothing further that could be done for the patient. In these earlier times, prognostication was a simpler process. The effectiveness of the therapeutic modalities in existence, including the few available surgical procedures, was so limited that patient prognosis was generally determined by the natural course of the disease. Prognostication was limited to simply patient follow-up. When the disease process accelerated or the patient's vital signs became unstable, it was clear to everyone that the patient was about to die. Nevertheless, the physician's affirmation frequently provided the patient and the family with a sense of closure and time to prepare both physically and emotionally for this unavoidable outcome.

Today the situation is quite different. With the many new advance in treatments, physicians gained the power to change the natural course of many diseases. With this newly acquired insight, the prognoses of those diseases improved as did the expectations about the curative power of medicine. The process became increasingly more complex to the point that many individuals believe that all diseases can be cured and that death represents a failure of some element of the health care system. Another change was the demise of prognostication.[4] Given this new knowledge, it became dangerous to attempt to convey a realistic patient prognosis. Instead physicians understandably chose to address everything more or less aggressively, whether or not the treatments and therapies provided were likely to alter patient prognosis. This has created a new problem of futile treatment. In today's litigious environment, physicians know that they are more likely to be held liable for these outcomes if they are perceived as doing too little rather than doing too much. An understanding of prognostication may place the physician back in control of patient care.

From the scientific point of view, patient prognosis depends on whether an individual can maintain a viable environment for their cells after they have sustained a pathophysiologic insult (figure 1.1).

---

[4] A. Ferrand, J. Poleksic, E. Racine, "Factors Influencing Physician Prognosis: A Scoping Review," *MDM Policy Pract* 7, no. 2 (2022), 23814683221145158.

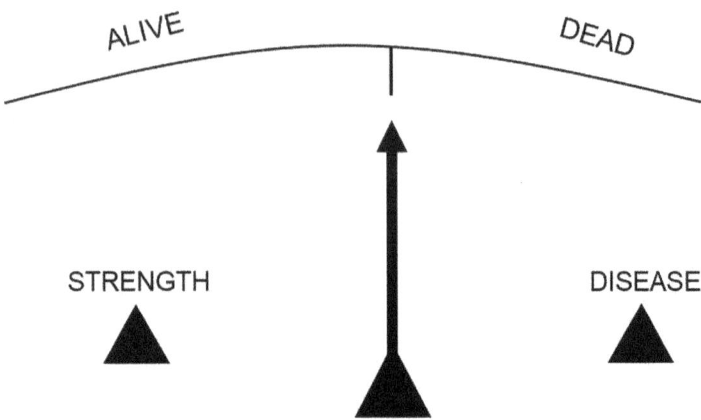

Figure 1.1. The balance between life and death

The many specialized cells found in the human body developed over millions of years of evolution and can thrive only in very specific environments that are defined by pH and osmolarity as well as oxygen, carbon dioxide, and nutrient concentrations, among other factors. Based on these needs and responses, single cells eventually differentiated and developed into organs with complex systems that maintain these specific environmental conditions. When these organs and systems fail irreversibly, death is the inevitable consequence.

In more specific terms, patient survival is based on the balance between the ability to maintain a viable environment, a concept known as "physiological strength," and the severity and overall impact of a pathophysiologic insult. In other words, the stronger the patient, the more he or she can survive this type of insult.

The process

No additional training will be needed to begin using prognostication methods beyond that currently provided to students in medical school and used in routine medical practice. The process simply requires the physician to perform an organized analysis of specific information and interpret the results. In other words, the physician needs to understand what information to consider, how to evaluate it, and how to determine its significance. Using this process, these findings can then be projected to predict the future of a given patient.

It is important to understand that this process is not substantially different from any other interactions between physicians and patients. Prognostication is designed to be practical and should not increase the burden of providing regular medical care. Furthermore, prognostication is not another complex and time-consuming mathematical tool. Prognostication is actually an intellectual process that a physician can follow when performing an evaluation and providing recommendations. For example, prognostication may lead to simple recommendations such as a change of diet or prescribing a single medication; it may also lead to complex recommendations, for example, surgical procedures, palliative care, or hospice.

The four essential steps of prognostication are as follows (figure 1.2):

- Analyze the patient data to determine a good or poor prognosis.
- Select the best plan of treatment for the patient based on this prognosis.
- Communicate the prognosis to the patient, family, or significant other, determine their wishes, and discuss recommended plan(s) of treatment and potential alternatives.
- Implement and follow the treatment plan with the understanding and agreement with the patient or the patient's family.

All patients are, of course, not the same. Therefore, treatments and recommendations need to be tailored to individual circumstances. Frequently, especially in younger patients who are most likely to be stronger and thus have a good prognosis, the benefit of treatment would clearly outweigh any of the risks involved. In these cases, the physician only goes through the intellectual steps of the process and explains the results to the patient and the patient's family. By contrast, if the patient is too sick or too weak and thus unlikely to receive benefits from specific treatments, the physician would need to go through all the stages of the process before reaching a decision.

To gain patient trust, the physician needs to have knowledge and experience as well as the ability to communicate and establish an empathetic relationship with the patient and the patient's family. This trust will be critical for any discussions of life and death matters that may determine the treatment of the patient.

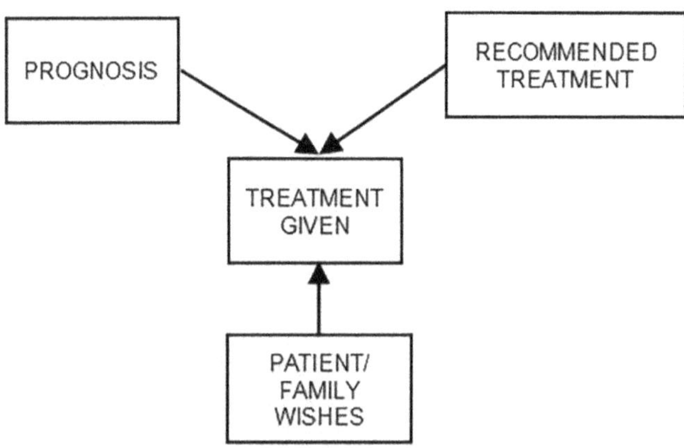

Figure 1.2. Four steps in patient prognostication

Prognostication may in some cases be stressful and emotionally involving for the physician.[5] This process requires time and preparation not only from the physician but also from the other disciplines and health care providers involved in patient care.

Physician perceptions of prognostication

Very few published studies focus on physician perceptions of prognostication.[4,6] The few that have been done suggest that physicians have created a culture in which prognostication is not well

---

[5] N. A. Christakis, MD; T. J. Iwashyna, AB, "Attitude and Self-reported Practice Regarding Prognostication in a National Sample of Interest." *Arch Intern Med*, vol. 158, November 23, 1998.

[6] C. Chu, N. White, P. Stone, "Prognostication in Palliative Care," *Clin Med (Lond)* 19, no. 4 (2019): 306–10.

received. Others report that physicians are concerned about the potentially negative consequences of prognostication, including

- distrust of physicians who try to prognosticate when caring for patients;
- incorrect prognoses, which may lead other physicians to think negatively about them;
- loss of patient trust in the physician who has provided a poor prognosis;
- presenting a patient with a poor prognosis, which may affect the quality of care received; and
- the patient giving up when provided with a poor prognosis.

While some of these concerns are undoubtedly real, the Patient Self-Determination Act (1990) states clearly that patients are the only ones with the right to make decisions about their medical care.[7] Thus, the patients need to know the truth about their prognosis and the possibilities of success of a given treatment, particularly if their prognosis is poor. Once the patient has been provided with adequate information, he or she should determine what kind of care might be preferred. As physicians and part of the team that provides care for the patient, we have the responsibility to inform our patients about their prognoses.

Benefits of prognostication

Not everything about prognostication is negative. Determining the prognosis of the patient in the regular practice of medicine has numerous benefits, including the following:

- It prevents unnecessary care.
- It prevents unnecessary suffering.

---

[7] D. Teoli, S. Ghassemzadeh, "Patient Self-Determination Act," updated August 29, 2022, in StatPearls (Internet) (Treasure Island, FL: StatPearls Publishing, January 2023), available from https://www.ncbi.nlm.nih.gov/books/NBK538297/.

- It helps to focus the treatment on what is important to patients.
- It helps patients and families to set realistic expectations.
- It gives patients and families time to prepare for the unavoidable.
- It decreases stress on patients, families, and caregivers.
- It makes economic sense.

With the rising number of older individuals in the population, physicians will be dealing with an increasing number of elderly patients who are frail and present with complex illnesses as they near the natural ends of their lives. The current standards of care that were developed for healthier younger individuals who are likely to live long enough to benefit from these treatments are not ideal for these older patients. Forced application of these standards of care on the elderly will generate unnecessary and potentially harmful futile care. Prognostication is a tool that can help physicians to navigate through the standardization and regulation of care that is currently imposed by the health care system. From the physician's perspective, prognostication is a task that requires patience, knowledge, experience, and understanding, as well as the ability to communicate and empathize with the patient. Prognostication brings the patient more benefits than the problems that result from implementing inappropriate care. Prognostication is an excellent practice that can be used to personalize patient treatment and will (albeit indirectly) permit the physician to regain control of patient care.

Prognostication is not the only change needed to solve the current crisis in medical practice. However, the use of this method will definitely improve the care of the patients and prevent painful, unwanted, and expensive *futile care*.

In the next chapters, the principles on which the process of prognostication is based will be reviewed. These subjects will be presented progressively, beginning with general principles, and following through to the use of this system at the bedside. In the next chapter, we will review the factors that under ordinary circumstances will determine the absolute maximum human life span.

CHAPTER 2

Maximum Potential Life Span

While humans are highly complex organisms with some unique attributes, they are part of the circle of life on earth. In this chapter, we discuss the human life span and what can (and cannot) be done to extend it past its natural limit. The median life expectancy in developed countries has increased dramatically in the past one hundred years. This has resulted in a profound increase in the fraction of the population currently greater than eighty-five years of age. We also discuss senescence, normal aging, and responses to disease and consider the impact of these conditions on the extent to which a patient can recover from a physiologic insult, *i.e.*, trauma or disease. Finally we introduce the concept of a metabolic equivalent of task or MET. This variable can be used as the basis of a quantitative evaluation of the amount of energy required to sustain basic life functions and for determining prognosis.

Objectives

The goals of this section are as follows:

- To review the factors that determine the human life span
- To understand the terminology and the changes associated with normal senescence and aging
- To educate physicians about the organs and organ systems that ultimately limit the human life span

Introduction

There is significant disagreement about what humans are, where they came from, and how long they can live. Contemporary science suggests that humans are both a part and a product of global order and that their biological systems are regulated by the same laws and principles as all other life forms. In other words, humans, by nature, are not very different from any other organisms living on earth. There are no fully unique components of the human body. Everything human also exists in a similar fashion to other natural organisms. These similarities exist in all dimensions, from the subatomic to the atomic, molecular, cellular, and physiological levels, and also include behavioral and social domains.

However, certain attributes are unique to humans. In general, humans exhibit a higher level of complexity and differentiation, particularly with respect to intelligence and self-awareness. These characteristics place humans at the top of the evolutionary order, as we currently understand it. However, despite the level of sophistication and knowledge humans have reached thus far, these traits do not permit them to alter their biological destiny in any substantial way. For now, humans still follow the same life cycle as do all other complex life forms, particularly those of mammals, which are understood to be the closest relatives of the human species. For example, the union of two parent cells is still required for human reproduction; this is followed by characteristic patterns of intrauterine and extrauterine growth and adulthood with the main focus on reproduction, followed by aging and finally dying.

The life cycles of various mammalian species differ considerably. For example, dogs and cats can live as long as fourteen years, and horses can survive for thirty years. The reasons underlying these differences are complex and remain poorly understood. In this chapter, we will review what is known about the human life span and the factors, organs, and organ systems that contribute to potential life expectancy.

Terminology

The terminology used to describe how long a human can live has not been fully standardized. As a result, different authors use various terms to express the same concept. Here I will define the terms used in this book to avoid confusion:

- The *life span* of an individual is the length of time that a person has lived. This can only be determined after an individual has died.
- The *average life span* is the overall average value of all individual life spans in a given population.
- The *median life expectancy* is the amount of time that 50 percent of the individuals in a given cohort born during the same time period might be expected to live.
- The *species maximum life span potential* is the maximum amount of time that an individual of a given species has lived. For humans, this value is 124 years.
- The *individual maximal life span potential* is the amount of time an individual could be expected to live under ideal conditions.
- *Additional life expectancy* is the number of additional years an individual could be expected to live upon the implementation of a specific change.

Other terms used will be defined if they are not self-explanatory.

Median life expectancy

Since the era of industrialization began, human life expectancy in developed countries has increased.

Table 2.1. Median life expectancy in the United States at birth (1900–2017)[8]

Year of birth	Both sexes	Male	Female
1900	47.3	46.3	48.3
1950	68.2	65.6	71.1
1960	69.7	66.6	73.1
1970	70.8	67.1	74.7
1980	73.7	70.0	77.4
1990	75.4	71.8	78.8
2000	76.8	74.1	79.3
2010	78.7	76.2	81.0
2014	78.9	76.5	81.3
2015	78.7	76.3	81.1
2016	78.6	76.1	81.1

The median life expectancy in the US has risen dramatically over the past one hundred years, from 47.3 years in 1900 to 76.8 years in 2000. Since hitting a high in 2014 with 78.9, the statistics have leveled or dipped slightly, until 2020 and 2021, with significant lowering in the wake of the global COVID-19 pandemic with median life expectancy dipping below the statistics in the year 2000. Similar figures have been reported by other developed countries. Many factors have contributed to these observations from 1900 to 2014. Improvements in sanitary and living conditions, the industrialization of agriculture, and advances in preventive and curative med-

---

[8] National Center for Health Statistics, 2017 Table 015, available at https://www.cdc.gov/nchs/hus/data-finder.htm?&subject=Life%20expectancy, "Life Expectancy at Birth, at Age 65, and gut Age 75, by Sex, Race, and Hispanic Origin: United States, Selected Years 1900–2016," available in PDF at https://www.cdc.gov/nchs/data/hus/2017/015.pdf. Data are based on death certificates and cover all races. Please note that median life expectancy in the US fell in 2020 and 2021 as a result of the worldwide COVID-19 pandemic. See https://www.cdc.gov/nchs/data/vsrr/vsrr023.pdf.

icine are most likely to be the main reasons underlying this profound increase. These improvements have allowed humans to live longer, as shown by specific statistics (table 2.1). More people are reaching old age and are approaching their maximum life span potential. The fastest-growing segment of the population includes individuals older than eighty-five years of age.

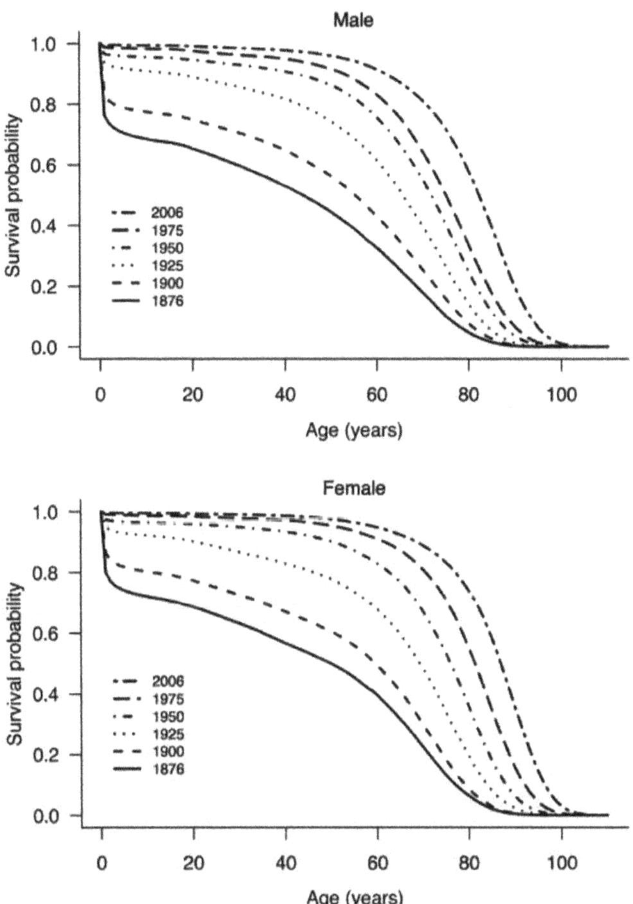

Figure 2.1. Percent survival probability divided by age and sex in the United States. Shown are data from the years 1876 to 2006. *E. Arias, National Vital Statistics Reports 54(14), April 19, 2006.* More information available here: https://www.cdc.gov/nchs/data/vsrr/vsrr023.pdf.

The graph shown in figure 2.1 represents the percentage of people surviving by age during intervals from the beginning, the middle, and the end of the twentieth century. The curves reveal that more people that were alive during 2006 reached old age compared to previous time intervals. However, the maximal life span has not changed significantly during this time and remains at ~100 years. This age will be used as the main reference point for the determination of the additional years of life expectancy and thus the prognoses of individual patients.

Factors determining the maximal life expectancy

Life expectancy is species-specific. The factors accounting for the differences between species are complex, poorly understood, and beyond the scope of this book. Here we will limit the discussion to maximal human life expectancy.

Changes in the environment have sculpted the nature of organic life today. While the special requirements of human cells, notably those associated with pH and osmolarity as well as oxygen and carbon dioxide concentrations, developed over millions of years, they were originally based on the nature of the environment at the beginning of life. Since that time, the changing environment has influenced organic life at all levels and has contributed to the determination of cell size, shape, and color, among other things. The environment ultimately determines which adaptations succeed, leading to organism survival, and likewise which organisms ultimately fail and die. As they are part of the same general order as all living beings, humans remain closely tied to their environment, which will also determine who will live and who will die on an individual basis.

Once humans developed self-awareness, they began to yearn for eternal life. There is abundant literature containing studies that attempt to unveil the secrets of longevity. This issue has been evaluated by many scientific disciplines, including but not limited to biochemistry, genetics, cellular biology, physiology, psychology, and sociology. While none of these studies have provided a pathway to eternal life, many have generated significant insight into these issues.

Many factors are involved in determining human life expectancy. Figure 2.2 illustrates the relationships between these factors. Most evidence suggests that the interaction between the individual genetic makeup (*i.e.*, genotype) and the environment is the main determinant of individual life expectancy.[9]

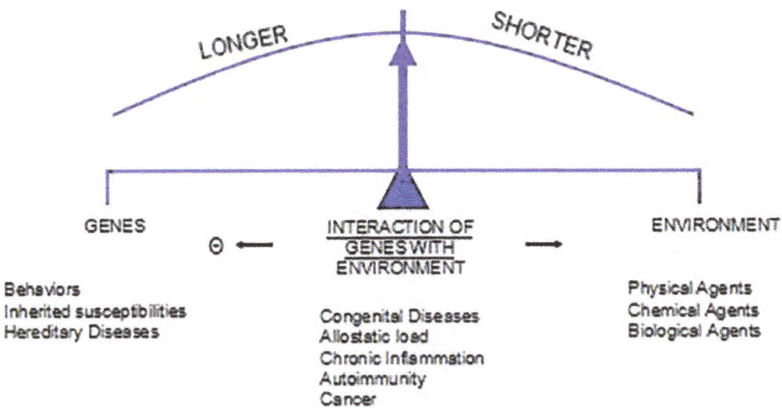

Figure 2.2. Factors that determine the human life span

Genes and genotypes are clearly significant contributory factors to human longevity. This issue has been considered by several authors, including Dr. M. J. Frederick, whose research focuses on individuals who have reached one hundred years of age or more. Results from his studies suggest that longevity results from a combination of specific genes and gene expression patterns.

One's genotype contributes to his/her particular characteristics and, consequently, the way he/she is likely to respond to the environment. Genes and gene expression also determine an individual's hereditary, including genetic abnormalities and susceptibilities to specific diseases. Counterproductive behaviors (*e.g.*, substance abuse), which have long been considered independent factors that limit longevity, are now understood to be at least in part genetically

---

[9] E. C. Prom-Wormley, J. Ebejer, D. M. Dick, M. S. Bowers, "The Genetic Epidemiology of Substance Use Disorder: A Review." *Drug Alcohol Depend* 180 (2017): 241–59.

determined. Several recent studies have highlighted the genetic predisposition for substance abuse.[8,10]

A single individual with a specific genotype will be confronted with environmental challenges from the moment of conception to the final minutes of life. Environmental exposures can include the impact of famines, natural catastrophes, war, toxins, and infections.

Interactions between genotype and environment determine the way an individual responds to the wear and tear of daily life. This interaction will also determine whether an individual will age normally or develop chronic diseases, for example, metabolic syndrome, hypertension, diabetes, arthritis, dementia, autoimmune disorders, or cancer.

In general terms, an individual is born with a genetically determined potential that will permit him or her to live for a specific number of years. The possibility of reaching this potential depends on the congruence of specific genes and gene expression patterns with the environment to which a person is exposed. This, of course, does not imply that all individuals living in a congruent environment could live one hundred years or more. The significant variability between genetic makeup and the environment ensures that the same results will not be achieved in all cases. In other words, an ideal combination of genes leading to prolonged survival in one environment at one time may not be a successful combination for someone in another situation. The individual who will live the longest is the one with a genetic makeup that is ideal for the "congruent" environment in which he/she is living.

Most of the gains in life expectancy reported over the past one hundred years are the result of two main factors. First, there has been a substantial modification of interactions between individuals with the environment, specifically, decreasing exposure to trauma, poor weather conditions, natural disasters, and unsanitary conditions, as well as a profound decrease in the physical demands associated with

---

[10] NIDA, "Genetics and Epigenetics of Addiction DrugFacts," August 5, 2019, retrieved from https://nida.nih.gov/publications/drugfacts/genetics-epigenetics-addiction on May 6, 2023.

regular daily living. The second reason relates directly to advances in medical sciences, which have collectively led to the prevention and control of infectious diseases, improvement in the management of many acute and chronic diseases, and stabilization of acutely ill patients. Most of the elderly individuals currently residing in assisted living facilities and nursing homes today would not have had the chance to reach such an advanced age ~100 years ago.

Senescence and normal aging

Older individuals routinely experience changes to both the body and mind. While some of these changes are considered part of the normal aging process and others are clearly due to disease, it is frequently difficult to differentiate between them. With the advances in medicine, changes that previously were considered normal aging now are identified as diseases. The best example of this phenomenon is the condition known as osteoporosis, in which bones become brittle, fragile, and susceptible to breakage. While this remains part of normal aging, it is now possible to treat this condition with specific medications. Other examples include diminished hearing, cataracts, and benign prostate hypertrophy, which are all amenable to specific treatment. What has not changed about growing older is the decrease in physical and physiological strength and consequently the ability to function.

Figure 2.3 documents the progressive decrease in function associated with advancing age. Parameters evaluated include decreases in the ability to care for oneself measured as deficits in activities of daily living (ADLs) and instrumental activities of daily living (IADLs).

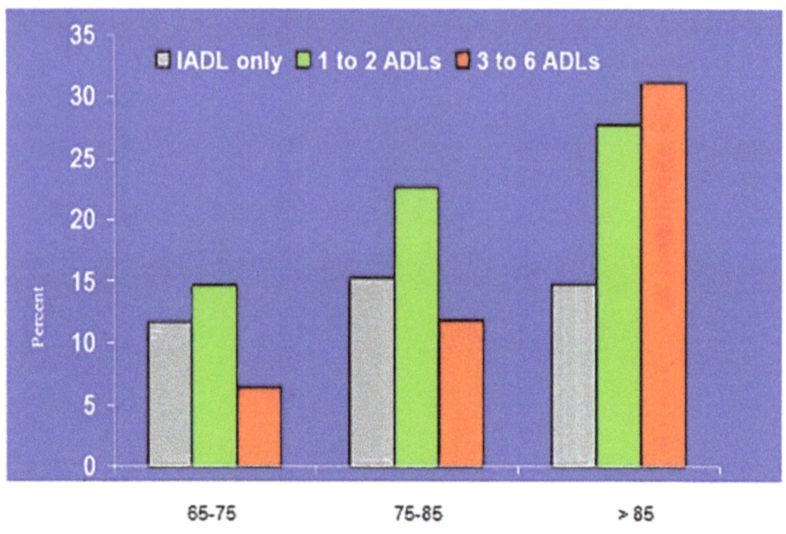

Figure 2.3. Percent of Medicare beneficiaries reporting difficulty with ADLs or IADLs by age group. The data shown are for the year 2002.

As an individual grows older, he or she may become weaker and more dependent on outside assistance.

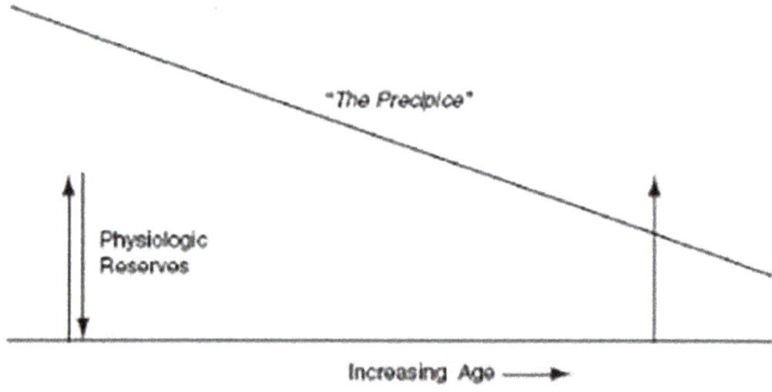

Figure 2.4. Graphical depiction of "the precipice." Reprinted from Cassel CK et al. *Geriatric Medicine. An Evidence Based Approach. 4th edition; Springer.*

This progressive decrease in strength and function is referred to as *the precipice* (figure 2.4).

For many years, scientists have questioned the concept of the precipice. The main focus of the dispute has been whether the downward slope is fully unavoidable or whether it relates specifically to (potentially avoidable or treatable) disease. A few well-designed studies were performed at the end of the twentieth century that addressed this specific question.[11] The authors of this study concluded that the downward slope was the result of two processes happening in a single individual at the same time. The first process, known as *senescence*, is the slowly progressive and unavoidable decrease in function. This process was amplified by one or more phenomena related to disease exposure, with the summation of both processes familiarly known as *aging*. One can understand this concept by considering the difference between the skin that is protected from the environment (*i.e.*, the lower back), which is affected only by senescence, compared to the skin exposed to the environment (*i.e.*, the face and arms), which also undergoes aging (*i.e.*, senescence and potential disease exposure). Another good example of this concept is the difference in life spans between animals of the same species who are living in the wild *versus* those that are domesticated and living in protected environments.

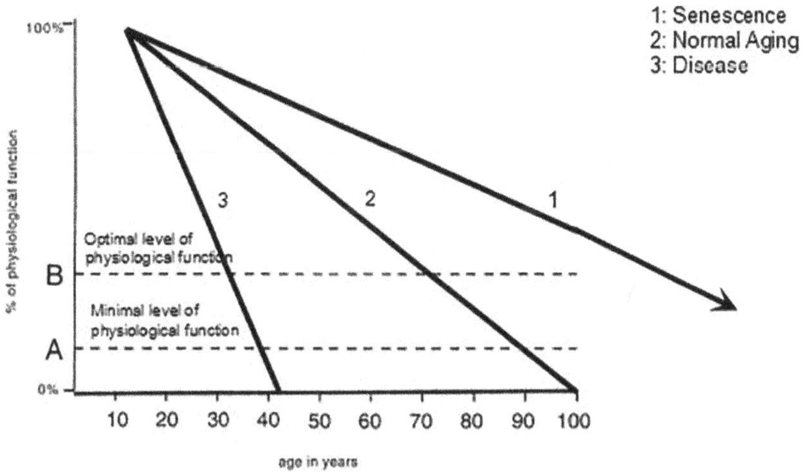

Figure 2.5. Decline in physiologic function with age

[11] E. Nakamura, "A Study on the Basic Nature of Human Biological Aging Processes Based upon a Hierarchical Factor Solution of the Age-Related Physiological Variables," *Mech Ageing Dev* 160 (1991): 153–170.

Three slopes with three different rates of aging are shown in figure 2.5. The uppermost line (no. 1) represents a hypothetical population with an ideal phenotype whose members are living in a perfectly congruent environment. By definition, these individuals experience only senescence. The only available real-life examples of this concept are the few exceptional elders that have lived to ~124 years, an age currently considered to represent the maximal potential life span for the human species. The middle line depicts the responses of a small group of individuals who have reached the maximal life span for the species, which, based on what was discussed previously, is ~100 years. The lowermost line is an extreme representation of a population in which most individuals develop chronic diseases or disabilities at a comparatively young age. Most of the patients who are under a physician's care regularly usually fall between the middle and lowermost lines. We will use this concept as the framework reference for performing prognostication in a given patient case.

Many members of the scientific community were also concerned about when (*i.e.*, at what age) the precipice begins. Some researchers believe that physical decline begins immediately upon growth cessation, which is approximately age twenty years. The problem with this assumption is that organs do not all cease growing at the same time. Other researchers believe that physical decline begins later. From the practical point of view, aging becomes measurable once an individual reaches an age of ~35 years.

The important point to understand is that death is the ultimate outcome, even for a hypothetical population responding only to senescence. Also, as shown in figure 2.5, the line representing the responses of individuals living up to one hundred years of age is understood to be the longest humans as a group can be expected to live. This will be used as a reference point for determining the life expectancy of our patients.

Table 2.2. Age-associated changes in human organs and organ systems

Item	Morphology	Function
General	Decreased height (vertebral compression and stooped posture secondary to increased kyphosis) Decreased weight (after age 80 in longitudinal studies) Increased fat-to-lean body mass ratio Decreased total body water	
Skin	Increased wrinkling Atrophy of the sweat glands	
Cardiovascular	Elongation and tortuosity of arteries, including the aorta Increased intimal thickening of the arteries Increased fibrosis of media of the arteries Sclerosis of the heart valves	Decreased cardiac output during exercise Decreased heart rate response to stress Decreased compliance of peripheral blood vessels
Kidney	Increased number of abnormal glomeruli Interstitial fibrosis	Decreased creatinine clearance Decreased renal blood flow Decreased maximum urine osmolality
Lung	Decreased elasticity Decreased activity of the cilia	Decreased forced vital capacity and forced expiratory volume Decreased maximal oxygen uptake Decreased cough reflex
Gastrointestinal tract	Decreased hydrochloric acid production Fewer taste buds	Slowed intestinal motility
Skeleton	Osteoarthritis Loss of bone structure	
Eyes	Arcus senilis Decreased pupil size Growth of lens	Decreased accommodation Hyperopia Decreased acuity Decreased color sensitivity

Hearing	Degenerative changes of ossicles Increased obstruction of the Eustachian tube Atrophy of cochlear hair cells Loss of auditory neurons	Decreased perception in high frequencies Decreased pitch discrimination
Immune system		Decreased T cell activity
Nervous system	Decreased brain weight Decreased cortical cell count	Increased motor response time Slower psychomotor performance Decreased intellectual performance Decreased complex learning Decreased hours of sleep Decreased hours of rapid eye movement (REM) sleep
Endocrine		Decreased triiodothyronine (T3) Decreased free (unbound) testosterone Increased insulin Increased norepinephrine Increased parathormone Increased vasopressin

Reprinted from Kane et al., *Essentials of Clinical Geriatrics*, 5th ed. (McGraw Hill Medical).

Thus, prognostication is a process that can be used to determine the position of an individual patient on these curves (*i.e.*, senescent only, normal aging, or disease) by systematically analyzing the pertinent patient information (see points A and B in figure 2.5). Consequently, one can determine the likelihood that a given patient will die in the near *versus* distant future. The risks and benefits of treatments can then be calculated according to the characteristics of each specific patient.

Organs and organ systems that determine the human maximal life span potential

While all organs and organ systems exhibit diminished function as they age, they do not all do so at the same rate. Some organs and organ systems age more rapidly than others. One good example of this point is the thymus, which is an immune organ that atrophies in humans at an early age. Another example is the ovaries which fail at the age ~45. Furthermore, some of the changes exhibited by the different organs and organ systems are more significant than others. The organs that decline and are the first to reach minimal levels of critical function should be the ones that determine when a healthy individual will undergo irreversible decline. This illustrates the basic principle that a chain is only as strong as its weakest link. Table 2.2 documents the changes in different organs that are anticipated with normal aging.

These changes are not of equivalent significance and can be divided into two groups, *i.e.*, changes that are and changes that are not the direct cause of death. Both groups are interrelated and dependent on one another, but they are not equivalent.

Among the changes that do not necessarily lead to death are those affecting the eyes, ears, central nervous system (CNS), skin, muscle, gastrointestinal tract, endocrine system, skeleton, and immune systems. These systems developed primarily as a means to enable an individual to interact with the environment. Organ-specific changes associated with normal aging leave elderly individuals at a disadvantage when interacting with the environment and leave them less tolerant to pathophysiologic insults and more susceptible to events that could result in death. However, this type of dysfunction will not ordinarily lead to the immediate death of a given individual.

Changes to organs and organ systems that directly control the microenvironment and maintain homeostasis, including the cardiovascular, respiratory, renal, and metabolic systems (also known as the "vital organs"), are more likely to lead to death. These organs regulate the microenvironment required by all cells and are responsible for maintaining appropriate pH; electrolyte concentrations; osmolarity;

concentrations of oxygen, carbon dioxide, and nutrients; and intercellular communication. Failure of any one of these organs or organ systems will result in death. The changes resulting from normal aging can result in the demise of an elderly patient.

There are no specific studies that focus on the significance of the different vital organs and their contributions to survival in response to normal aging. The evidence suggesting their crucial role remains circumstantial and based on projections of what has been considered by several authors as the normal decrease of function due to aging.

The cardiovascular system includes the heart, blood vessels, microcirculation, and lymphatic systems. This system maintains the microenvironment needed by viable cells by delivering oxygen, nutrients, and intercellular messages and also by removing carbon dioxide and waste products. The cardiovascular system is complex; there are no readily usable and practical tests of cardiac function and reserve available to those engaged in routine medical practice. To date, the best option available in this setting is the stress test. This test measures the function and reserves of the system by quantitatively evaluating the capacity to deliver oxygen during maximal exercise (maximal oxygen consumption), as measured in metabolic equivalents of task (METs). One (1) MET is the amount of oxygen consumed by a healthy forty-year-old man at rest, *i.e.*, the minimal amount of energy produced by a body to keep all systems running. A normal healthy individual at the end of the period of growth who is not participating in athletic training should be able to produce with thirteen METs. When the intensity of the exercise increases higher than 60 percent of the individual's total maximal capacity, the metabolism progressively changes from aerobic to anaerobic, which limits the ability to exercise. Most people attempt to maintain their level of activity to ~50–60 percent of their maximal oxygen consumption.

Table 2.3. The veterans-specific activity questionnaire

Before beginning your treadmill test today, we need to estimate what your usual limits are during daily activities. The following is a list of activities that increase in difficulty as you read down the page. Think carefully, then underline the first activity that, if you performed it for a period of time, would typically cause fatigue, shortness of breath, or chest discomfort, or otherwise cause you to want to stop. If you do not normally perform a particular activity, try to imagine what it would be like if you did.

1 MET: Eating; getting dressed; working at a desk

2 METs: Taking a shower; shopping; cooking; walking down eight steps

3 METs: Walking slowly on a flat surface for one or two blocks; doing moderate amounts of work around the house like vacuuming, sweeping the floors, or carrying in groceries

4 METs: Doing light yard work, i.e., raking leaves, weeding, sweeping, or pushing a power mower; painting; light carpentry

5 METs: Walking briskly; social dancing; washing the car

6 METs: Playing nine holes of golf, carrying your own clubs; heavy carpentry; mowing lawn with a push mower

7 METs: Carrying 60 lbs.; performing heavy outdoor work, i.e., digging, spading soil, etc.; walking uphill

8 METs: Carrying groceries upstairs; moving heavy furniture; jogging slowly on flat surface; climbing stairs quickly

9 METs: Bicycling at a moderate pace; sawing wood; jumping rope (slowly)

10 METs: Briskly swimming; bicycling up a hill; jogging 6 mph

11 METs: Carrying a heavy load (i.e., a child or firewood) up two flights of stairs; cross-country skiing; bicycling briskly and continuously

12 METs: Running briskly and continuously (level ground, 8 mph)

13 METs: Performing any competitive activity, including those that involve intermittent sprinting; running competitively; rowing competitively; bicycle racing

The findings presented in table 2.3 detail the number of METs required for different activities. The cardiovascular literature, most notably the studies related to indications for cardiac transplant, documents the close correlation between cardiovascular fitness and the ability to function.

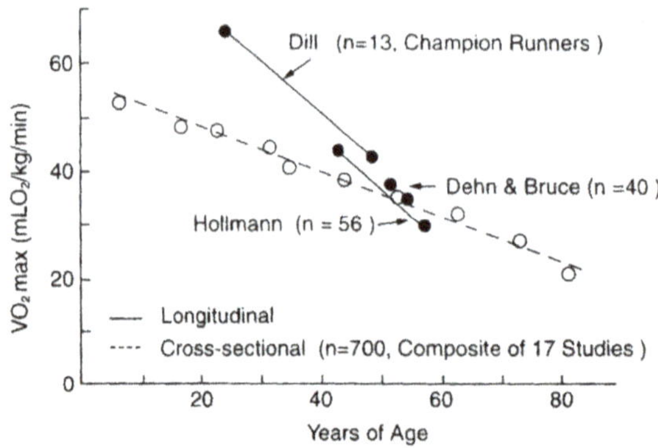

Figure 2.6. Changes in oxygen consumption that occur with aging. *Reprinted from Hazard et al.,* Principles of Geriatric Medicine and Gerontology, *5th ed. (McGraw Hill Companies, Inc.).*

The maximal oxygen consumption initially increases during development and then progressively decreases with age. Figure 2.6 shows the changes in oxygen consumption as a function of age, measured as mL oxygen/kg/min (n.b.: one MET is equivalent to ~3.6 mL oxygen/kg/min). The findings reveal a steady decline that was more rapid in the longitudinal compared to the cross-sectional studies. These differences might be due to variations in these types of studies.

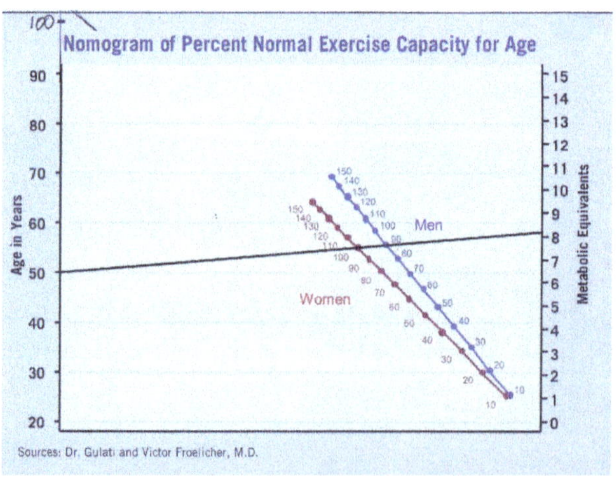

Figure 2.7. Percent of normal exercise capacity by age

Routine exercise and training increase the number of METs an individual can perform. The findings presented in figure 2.7 document the number of METs a male or female can perform (measured in percentages) based on his/her age and state of fitness. The findings shown in this figure also document that the older the person, the more modest the improvement in METs and, thus, the more modest the improvement in fitness.

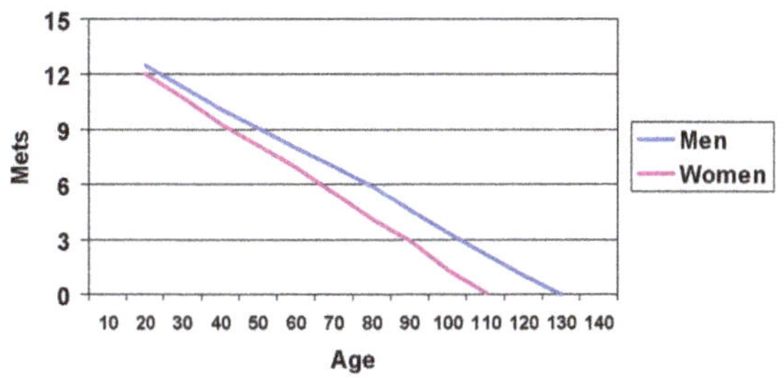

Figure 2.8. Theoretical METS at each age. Findings are based on data shown in figure 2.7.

The graphic shown in figure 2.8 was prepared using the data presented in figure 2.7, based on the premise that an individual has to produce a minimum of one MET to stay alive. The graphic shows that a fully (100 percent) physically fit woman could live up to 105 years and a fully physically fit man, up to 125 years. Interestingly, these numbers approximate the species-specific maximal life span potential that we discussed at the beginning of the chapter.

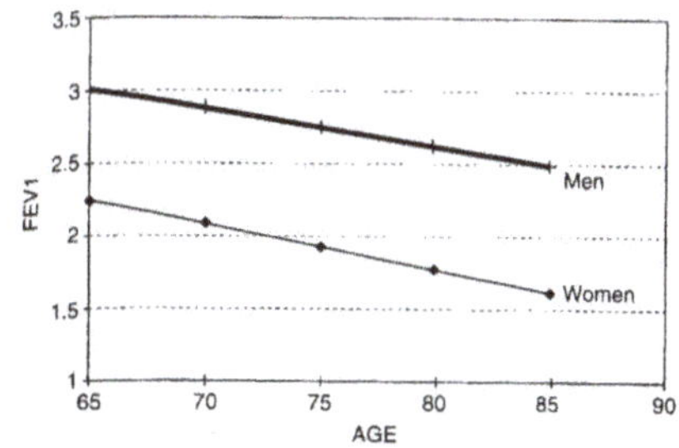

Figure 2.9. Decline in forced expiratory volume in one second (FEV1) with age. *Reprinted from Hazard et al., Principles of Geriatric Medicine and Gerontology, 5th Edition.*

The data for the respiratory system is not as clear as for the cardiovascular system (figure 2.9). If we consider the minimal amount of respiratory function needed to be alive and the changes due to normal aging (1 L of FEV1), this will be achieved in 110 years for women and nearly 170 years for men. One hundred and ten years is the approximate maximal life span potential for women.

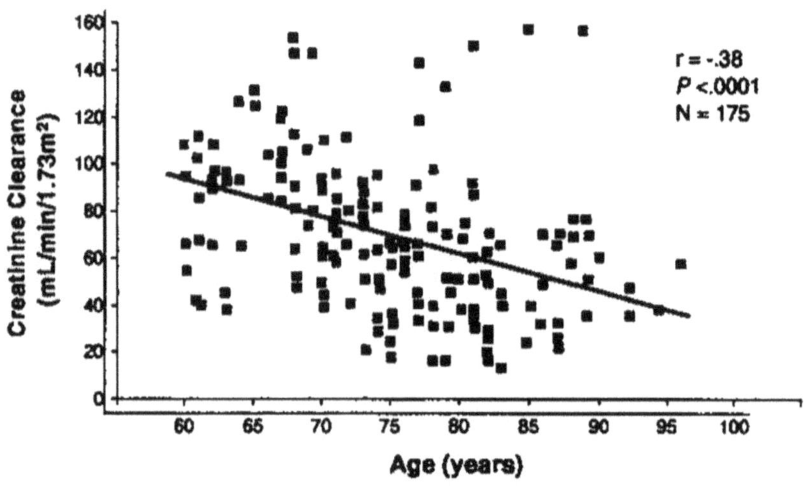

Figure 2.10. Decline in creatinine clearance with age. *Reprinted from B. G. Pollock et al. Psychopharmacol. Bull. 1995; 31:327.*

The projections based on renal (kidney) function are somewhat more complicated (figure 2.10). In some individuals, renal function declines only minimally with aging, while others respond with dramatic decreases over the years for no definitive reason. If we consider a creatinine clearance of 15 mL/min/1.73 m² as the minimal renal function compatible with life in the absence of dialysis, an average normal elderly person would reach this point at an age of approximately 120 years. This calculation places the kidney just above the level of importance of the respiratory systems and cardiovascular systems; 120 years is certainly longer than the maximal life span.

Finally, we consider the metabolic system. While the contributions of this system are not very well-defined or understood, they are of significant importance to life and health. The metabolic system regulates the nutritional aspects of all cells by controlling the metabolism of carbohydrates, proteins, and fats as well as the detoxification of exogenous and endogenous substances, among other benefits. The liver is the best-known of the metabolic organs, followed closely by the pancreas. There are no clinically useful tests to measure liver function and reserves. Tests of prealbumin, albumin, ammonia, and glucose levels together with prothrombin time are strong indicators of the health or failure of the metabolic system, although these tests do not measure metabolic reserves.

Every organ and system in the body undergoes functional decline because of changes resulting from normal aging. The changes are important in several different ways. Some of these changes do not result in death directly, although they do place individuals at a disadvantage and more susceptible to catastrophic health events. Changes in the function of cardiovascular, respiratory, renal, and metabolic systems will limit the life span of an elderly person even in circumstances associated with normal aging.

In our society, in which many believe that all diseases can be cured, the concept of unavoidable death due to old age is virtually incomprehensible. Physicians providing care for these individuals are confronted on the one hand with nonexistent or irrelevant standards of care and current practices that do not meet patient needs. It is important to understand the boundaries of human longevity and to be able to identify normal aging so that abnormal responses can be identified and treated. Also a more complete understanding of these changes will help physicians and their patients to set realistic expectations based on individualized life expectancy and avoid futile care.

Summary

The process of prognostication will help the physician to chart the patient as accurately as possible on the curve representing physical decline. Once a prognosis has been determined, the physician can then generate an estimate of the patient's future life span and develop a treatment plan according to the particular patient's situation.

Having a clear understanding of the reasons underlying limitations of the human life span will make it easier to appreciate the factors that abbreviate this potential. In the next chapter, we will explore the reasons this happens and review our current understanding of specific markers and their associated statistical significance when identifying a patient with a shorter-than-average life expectancy.

CHAPTER 3

Factors and Markers of a Reduced Potential Life Span

Despite increases in the median life span, many recent medical advances do not lead to improved health and longevity in all patients. In this chapter, we review the factors that lead to differences in individual life spans. This can be understood mechanistically as the extent to which a given individual can sustain or recover homeostasis after a pathophysiologic insult. The degree to which this can be achieved depends directly on the patient's reserves of physiological strength and the strength and duration of various internal and external challenges and stressors. Physicians need to have an in-depth understanding of this critical balance which is essential for determining patient prognosis and implementing suitable therapies and management strategies that are appropriate for individual geriatric patients.

Objectives

The goals of this section are as follows:

- To review the concepts of physiological strength, homeostasis, and organ failure
- To identify factors that determine the response to disease
- To discuss the importance of the environment
- To examine how those factors change with age
- To provide an overview of the markers of reduced life expectancy

Introduction

The existence of life, as we know it, is the result of interactions between the environment and factors that determine the existence of organic matter over many centuries. Based on millions of years of evolution, organisms have developed characteristics that permit them to survive in a changing environment. Specific environmental characteristics are needed to promote growth, appropriate function, and reproduction to continue species persistence and the cycle of life. In this context, humans are not very different from most other organisms. Similar to their single-celled counterparts, humans need to interact with and are largely dependent on a specific given environment.

The experiences of developed countries reveal that while advances in the control of the environment may extend longevity, living with full access to food, physical comforts, advanced medical care, and work that requires less physical output is not necessarily conducive to better health. Some humans have been able to find the ideal equilibrium with the environment and reach the maximal life span for the species, which is ~100 years; an occasional individual reaches the maximal life span potential for the species, which is 124 years.

With these statements in mind, together with the factors that determine the maximal life span potential that were discussed in the previous chapter, we are now ready to consider what may prevent an individual from reaching his/her maximal life span potential.

The findings presented in figure 3.1 represent the factors that will ultimately determine the life span of a particular individual, based on the fact that survival is the result of the interaction between the physiological strength of the individual and the severity of the challenge to be confronted.[12]

---

[12] K. T. Patton, G. A. Thibodeau, *The Human Body in Health and Disease*, 7th ed. (Elsevier—Health Sciences Division, 2017).

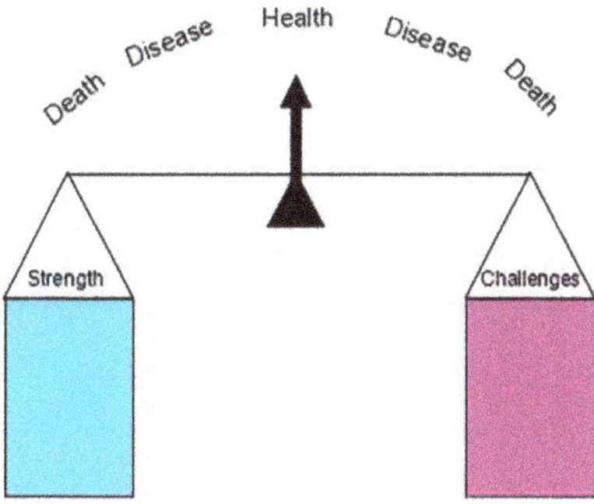

Figure 3.1. Factors that determine individual life span

Physiological strength

Physiological strength is the term used to describe the capacity of an organism to survive a pathophysiologic attack. In scientific terms, physiological strength is the ability of the individual to maintain the microenvironment needed by the cells and to maintain homeostasis, while undergoing attack by insults produced by the environment. Physiological strength will determine the ability of an individual to survive this type of onslaught.

Currently there are no direct methods that can be used to quantify individual physiological strength. However, the function and reserves of the organs and systems can be quantified and can be used to determine the physiological strength of the cardiovascular, respiratory, renal, and metabolic systems.

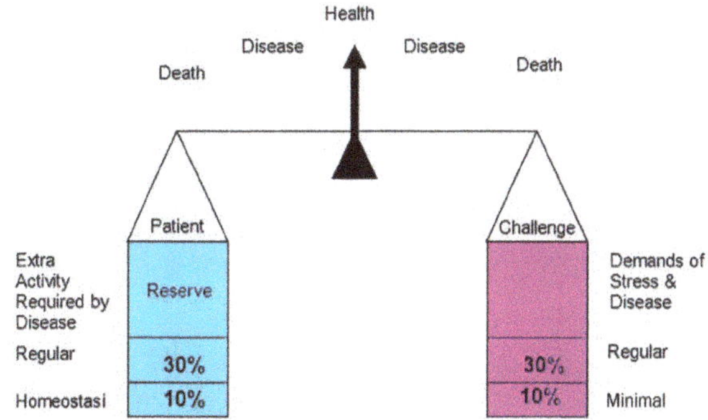

Figure 3.2. Graphical depiction of physiological strength

The illustration shown in figure 3.2 represents the nature of the physiological strength of an individual under normal circumstances. A healthy young person uses 10 percent or less of their total physiological capacity to maintain the ideal microenvironment. Another 30–40 percent is used to keep up with the demands of the activities of daily living (ADLs), except for those individuals performing physical work. These individuals will use a larger percentage of their capacity depending on the demands of the job. The remainder of the unused strength is the *reserve*, which is the cushion that the organism has available if it needs to deal with situations of stress or disease. As we can see, the body only uses a small amount of physiological strength to maintain the critical microenvironment.

Homeostasis

Homeostasis has been defined as a regulatory mechanism used by biological systems to maintain the internal stability necessary for survival and for adjusting to any internal or external threats. When homeostasis succeeds, life continues; when it fails, the individual dies.[13]

Vital organs and organ systems work together to maintain homeostasis and a viable microenvironment for their constituent cells. While these organs and organ systems have their own regulatory and compensatory mechanisms, they also interact with and depend on one another. When an organ suffers damage, the resulting dysfunction will affect that particular system first. Depending on the severity of the insult, there will be a significant impact on the function of organs and organ systems and, eventually, the entire organism, potentially resulting in death.

The body responds to insults on several levels. Beginning at the lowest level of complexity, the cells within a given organ can respond to changes in the environment. The individual cells have mechanisms that permit them to compensate for significant changes in pH, osmolarity, and oxygen saturation, among others. Working together,

---

[13] L. R. Johnson, *Essential Medical Physiology*, 3rd ed. (Elsevier, 2003), 4.

groups of cells can control regional blood flow, thereby managing local conditions and their environment. At a higher level, the different organs and organ systems can cooperate to control function as required. Among these systemic responses, physicians are familiar with shock, which is the deviation of blood flow toward the heart, lungs, and brain in response to dire conditions, for example, severe blood loss. At the highest level, humans can use their intuition and intelligence to support their own survival by maneuvering to avoid potential insults or injury.

As a final level of protection, certain organs can regenerate. After they are fully developed, many organs maintain a pool of primordial cells (*i.e.*, stem cells) that can be used to replace functional cells lost to injury and death as part of the wear and tear from day-to-day life. The capacity for regeneration becomes more active in response to an increase in cellular damage. However, the more specialized cells and organs, such as those in the nervous system, heart, skeletal muscle, and kidney, are less likely to be capable of full reconstruction and self-replacement. Frequent challenges to homeostasis that remain within the physiological range can result in organ hypertrophy or hyperplasia, thereby increasing physiological function and reserve. It is not clear whether this temporary increase will reduce the life span of the cells by using up their capacity to divide and compromising the life span of the organ. Nonetheless, the ability to regenerate clearly decreases with aging.

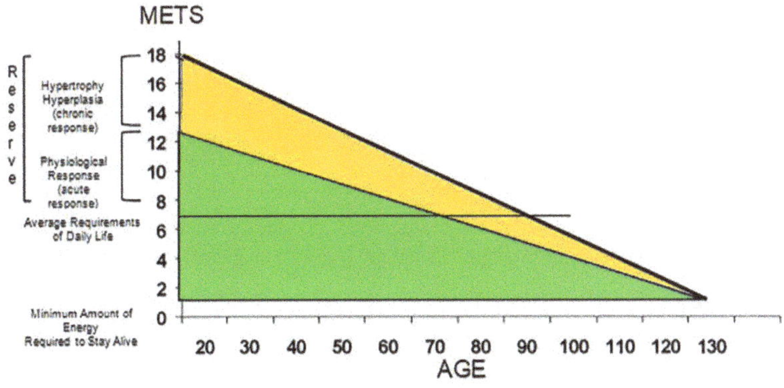

Figure 3.3. Senescence and aging in a hypothetical healthy population

The maximal physiological capacity as well as the capacity to undergo hypertrophy or hyperplasia stabilizes at the age of full development (figure 3.3). After that, both processes undergo a progressive decline in response to normal aging until the capacity to recover homeostasis has been irretrievably compromised and the individual dies.

When homeostasis has been threatened, the body responds with overlapping mechanisms of compensation based on an individual's physiological strength, remaining reserves, and the severity of the challenge. In nonlethal situations, the initial response in a normal and otherwise healthy individual is based on his or her physiological reserve. For example, most physicians will be familiar with the characteristic increase in heart and respiratory rates that can be easily detected in response to exercise, stress, or infection. If the initial responses are insufficient, other physiological changes can occur, for example, a shift of electrolytes into or out of the cell. This can result in an acid-based imbalance, the accumulation of intracellular osmotic substances in the cell, and a biochemical shift in hemoglobin leading to the release of oxygen, among other responses. If the challenge is strong or persistent enough to cause tissue damage, cell and tissue repair mechanisms are activated.

Organ damage

Challenges that extend beyond physiological reserves can accelerate cell destruction and activate organ repair processes. By contrast, while challenges resulting in only minimal damage will allow the system to maintain function and the microenvironment, each episode will decrease the life span and reserve of the target organ. Repeated episodes will decrease the reserves of the organ to the point at which it can no longer maintain its microenvironment. With more severe challenges, the function stabilizes at a lower level; if the organ can be repaired, its function could be improved. As illustrated in both scenarios, if the system cannot be repaired to the extent necessary to maintain the microenvironment, overall survival will depend on the ability and the time allotted for the cells to adapt to the new disequilibrium. A good example of this phenomenon is the tolerance to hypoxia that develops in patients with long-standing chronic obstructive pulmonary disease. These patients, who have had a long time to adapt to reduced oxygenation, can be compared to those unable to tolerate hypoxia that develops in response to acute pneumonia. In all cases, when one system is failing, the others try to adapt so that they can tolerate the lower level of function. Of note, this secondary decrease in function might be reversible. An example of this response is the improvement in cardiac function observed after a renal transplant. This result suggests that the other organs have adapted but have not lost their entire physiological reserve. These interactions are complex and cannot be measured directly. Thus, it can be quite difficult to determine the impact of these findings on the life span of a given patient.

From the patient's perspective, these responses and interactions ultimately translate into a state of health or illness. Health has been defined as physical, mental, and social well-being.[14] This definition includes three dimensions, as health can be measured at cellular, psychological, and functional levels and based on one's ability to interact with the environment. These are the same dimensions used by physicians to assess patient health and well-being as part of the general practice of medicine.

By contrast, disease has been defined as a condition that results from abnormalities of body structures or functions that prevent the body from maintaining homeostasis, which keeps us alive and healthy.[15] This term is universally understood and used as the basis of the evolution of the health care system. Recent advances in medical care have been based largely on research into how specific disease processes developed and ways that might be used to treat them. Most physicians receive training that has focused on ways to diagnose and treat these diseases. Furthermore, the current reimbursement system in the US and specific quality measures are also based on these same

---

[14] P. Thibodeau, "What Is Disease: The Human Body in Health," December 8, 2005, 4th ed. (Elsevier Mosby).

[15] R. Johnson, "Essentials of Medicine Physiology," 3rd ed. (Elsevier 2003), 4.

concepts. Knowledge and understanding of the natural course of a disease is an essential part of the practice of medicine and also of prognostication. Without this knowledge, a physician will be unable to determine whether a specific therapy provided to a patient has made a significant difference or whether the responses observed were simply the results of the natural course of the disease.

Factors that determine the ability of an individual to survive disease

Excellent health is the result of an ideal equilibrium (congruence) between the strength of the individual and challenges from the environment. An imbalance in this equilibrium challenges the individual's ability to maintain homeostasis, overworks the system, and reduces the individual's potential life span.

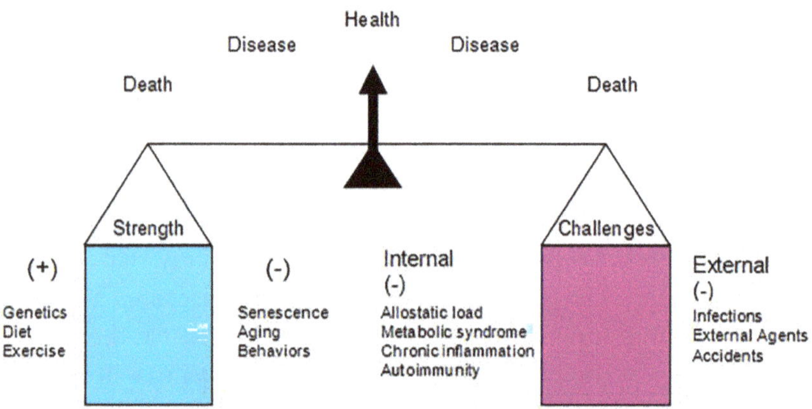

Figure 3.4. Factors that determine survival in response to disease

The illustration shown in figure 3.4 represents the factors that determine one's ability to survive disease; interestingly these are the same factors that determine life expectancy. These factors are classified as having a positive or negative impact on survival, physiological strength, and severity of challenge.

One's genetic makeup, or genotype, is one of the factors that can have a generally positive impact on physiological strength. However, this factor can work in both ways. As was mentioned earlier, longevity is the result of a combination of having some genes and not having others. While some individuals are born with genes and gene expression patterns that promote longevity, others are born with hereditary diseases or the susceptibility to develop specific diseases over time. Apart from the very few genetic diseases currently believed to be directly amenable to gene therapy, the benefits of assessing these genetic factors are currently limited to the identification of genetically determined diseases and susceptibilities, including responses to some therapies and organ transplantation. However, the situation is different when discussing diet and exercise. Most evidence suggests that individuals who exercise regularly and consume low-calorie diets develop metabolic markers similar to those of individuals known to have comparatively long life spans. These specific changes most likely result in increased physiological strength and the ability to survive over time.

The factors that tend to have a negative impact on physiological strength include senescence, aging, and counterproductive behaviors.[16] As shown in figure 3.4, these factors will erode physiological strength over time. Senescence leads to a slow depletion of physiologic reserves over time until they are completely gone. When this happens, one's ability to maintain the microenvironment is compromised, and the individual will die due to old age. The changes produced by disease (aging) and counterproductive behaviors will accelerate the decline and decrease an individual's life span. The demise typically results from the inability to maintain the microenvironment when confronted with a challenge (for example, an infection or trauma) that overwhelms one's physiological strength.

The challenges involved in maintaining homeostasis can be classified into two categories: internal and external.

---

[16] R. Andersen, J. F. Newman, "Societal and Individual Determinants of Medical Care Utilization in the United States," *Milbank Mem Fund Q Health Soc* 51, no. 1 (1973):95–124.

Internal challenges are the result of the body's efforts to maintain homeostasis. The effect is known as the allostatic load, which is defined as the cumulative physiological burden exacted on the body due to attempts to adapt to life. Numerical measures of allostatic load predict cardiovascular disease as well as declines in physiological and cognitive function and mortality.[17] The overall impact of the allostatic load depends on genetically determined responses and the cumulative frequency and severity of one's personal challenges. Each person responds differently to challenges, even ones that are similar to one another. The physiological dysfunction resulting from an increase in the allostatic load is manifested in clinical terms by metabolic syndrome, hypertension, vascular disease, and diabetes, along with the consequences of these disorders. Cancer, allergic disorders, and autoimmune diseases represent another large group of diseases that result from interactions with the environment. These diseases will also erode physiological reserve and limit the potential life span potential of an affected individual.

External challenges tend to be more familiar and include trauma, infections, and toxic environments, among others. In general terms, an individual can survive only if the challenge permits one's compensatory mechanisms to restore the microenvironment to a viable level (figure 3.1).

The damage one sustains in response to an external insult or challenge depends on three specific characteristics: speed, intensity, and duration. The speed of a given challenge is important because it determines whether one's body will be capable of responding, for example, in cases associated with traumatic events. Emergency physicians are familiar with the differential damage that can be induced by a low-speed *versus* a high-speed motor vehicle crash. Similarly rapid loss of blood secondary to a traumatic event will be more damaging than the loss of the same amount of blood at a slower rate, for example, due to a gastrointestinal bleed. Similarly heart damage resulting

---

[17] D. Bialostozky, M. Levya, T. Villareal, et al., "Myocardial Perfusion and Ventricular Function Assessed by SPECT and Gated-SPECT in End-Stage Renal Disease Patients before and after Renal Transplant," *Arch Med Res* 38, no. 2 (2007): 227–233.

from slow but progressive obstruction of a coronary artery will have less of an acute impact than sudden obstruction of an otherwise normal vessel. These same principles regarding the speed of the external insult apply to other processes, including infections and the ingestion of toxins.

The intensity of the insult will also be a major factor in determining whether one's response will be sufficient to recover homeostasis. The more intense the insult, the greater the damage; this reduces the likelihood of returning to a viable state of equilibrium. The intensity of the insult may be significant in response to trauma or exposure to extreme or toxic environments, including excessive heat, cold, sun, radiation, and toxins, among others. The intensity of the insult is also important in response to infectious disease processes. In this scenario, the intensity of the insult might depend on the number of microorganisms involved and the aggressiveness of a specific pathogen.

The duration of the attack is also a clinically important factor. The longer the exposure, the more damage one is likely to sustain. This characteristic plays a significant role not only in trauma and exposure to toxic environments but also when considering the impact of chronic diseases such as hypertension, metabolic syndrome, diabetes mellitus, autoimmunity, cancer, and chronic infections.

In clinical practice, the interactions among these three characteristics—the speed, intensity, and duration of the insult—will determine the extent and severity of the damage and the likelihood that one can recover to maintain a viable microenvironment. These interactions will thus have a substantial impact on the likelihood of survival.

Markers of a reduced life expectancy

For many decades, researchers have sought ways to predict when an individual may be nearing death. The issue has been examined from many different angles, from the biochemical to the sociological realm. While many indicators have been identified, no single marker can predict the accurate time of death. The human body is complex and resilient and has numerous compensatory mechanisms. The time of death is by its nature a moving target. Recent advances in medical care, for example, home ventilators, hemodialysis, and heart support devices to name a few, as well as the technological advances featured in hospital-based intensive care units, have collectively changed the significance of many of the markers that had previously been used to predict death. As we learn more about specific diseases, the more difficult it may become to differentiate between the effects of senescence *versus* aging.

Most of the markers used to identify patients with reduced life expectancy, for example, changes in one's complete blood count, liver function tests, serum uric acid, and basic metabolic panel, among others, are based on the premise that normal aging will not result in any specific change in these values from those considered within normal limits for younger individuals. The concept is appropriate in the sense that the normal values represent the normal microenvironment. Changes in these values imply a failure of the compensatory mechanisms and stabilization of the system at a lower level of functioning.

The literature on markers of reduced life expectancy is extensive. A detailed review of these findings is beyond the scope of this book. Considering the complexity of the issue, we will focus on the markers used in regular clinical practice that have been divided into categories pertinent to our discussion.

These categories include the following:

- Demographics
- Social dysfunction
- Function
- Aging
- Dysfunction of vital organs and immune system
- Allostatic load
- Specific disease
- Symptoms

Demographics

Age markers can be described as either chronological or physiological. Chronological age refers to the number of years that an individual has lived based on his or her date of birth. Physiological age is a concept used to describe how an individual compares to the standards for the decline in physiological strength due to normal aging (figure 3.4). There is significant individual variability based on these two parameters. It is not unusual to see younger individuals who are ill and appear to be older than their chronological age. Likewise many well-elderly individuals appear younger than would be expected given their chronological ages. While chronological age is the most significant predictor of years of life expectancy for the healthy elderly because they follow the predicted curve, the situation is less clear for those who have aged prematurely. This is because of the mismatch between their chronological and physiological ages and the fact that they do not follow the curve. While physiological age seems to be a better predictor of additional years of life in these patients, they will always be positioned above the standard curve.

Gender is also another predictor of mortality. It is well-known that women live longer than men. However, apart from its role as an indicator for population studies, analyses, and projections of public health issues, male *versus* female sex is not a very helpful parameter for determining the prognosis of an individual patient.

Social dysfunction

One of the main factors determining survival is the capacity for interactions with one's environment. Conversely the failure to interact successfully is an excellent indicator of reduced life expectancy. This has been documented by the results of the Andersen Model of Outcome Predictors study.[18] In this study, Andersen identified

---

[18] R. Andersen, J. Newman, "Andersen Study: Societal and Individual Determinants of Medical Care Utilization Milbank Memorial Fund," *Quarterly*, vol. 51 (Winter 1973): 95–124.

several characteristics leading to a reduced life expectancy, including an extreme need for personal control (*i.e.*, refusal to accept help), poor behavior, self-rated decreased health, prior hospitalizations, and number of days in the hospital. He also identified characteristics leading to a longer life expectancy, including greater social activity, a high body mass index, and living in a certified nursing home or a nursing home with a high caregiver-to-patient ratio.

Function

As part of one's ability to interact with the environment, a reduced function has been identified as an excellent marker for reduced life expectancy.[19] The significance of these findings is based on the noted correlation between cardiovascular reserve and function. This decrease in function is typically measured by one's ability to perform ADLs and IADLs. An inability to perform these basic functions has been identified as an excellent marker for poor prognosis and is also a predictor of a reduced life expectancy.

Aging

Based on the evidence reviewed thus far, physiologic changes associated with normal aging will eventually lead to death. Thus, any test results that identify normal or accelerated aging processes may be taken as indicators of a reduced life expectancy. Several changes associated with aging that have been considered in this context include decreased hearing or vision, unexplained weight loss, loss of height, decreases in mental capacity and processing, and the reduced ability to walk and maintain equilibrium, among many other factors.

---

[19] D. Bialostozky, "Myocardial Perfusion and Ventricular Function Assessed by SPECT and Gated-SPECT in End-Stage Renal Disease Patients before and after Renal Transplant," *Arch. Med-Res*, February 2007, vol. 38, no. 2: 227–3.

Dysfunction of vital organs and immune system

While changes that result from the normal aging process tend to be good indicators of a reduced life expectancy, markers documenting organ and system dysfunction (*e.g.*, cardiovascular, respiratory, renal, hematological, neurological, and metabolic systems) do not predict imminent death. However, these markers are reliable predictors of premature aging and a decreased life expectancy. The most thoroughly documented of these clinical markers include anemia associated with chronic diseases, hypoalbuminemia, and a decreased glomerular filtration rate. Other significant markers include hyponatremia, hyperbilirubinemia, leukocytosis, lymphopenia, hyperuricemia, proteinuria, persistently elevated levels of brain natriuretic peptide, and prolonged prothrombin time. Overall, the results of any clinical test that highlights an inability to maintain an appropriate microenvironment, for example, severe metabolic or respiratory acidosis, high lactic acid levels, significant changes in osmolarity, hypoxemia, and increased or decreased vascular resistance, are excellent markers and predictors of imminent death.

Allostatic load

This syndrome has been studied extensively and includes abnormalities in the lipid profile, insulin resistance, and dysregulated levels of adrenocorticotrophic hormone (ACTH) and catecholamines in the blood. As a group, these markers represent an inability to handle stress. The most significant contributors to this category are hypertension, obesity, atherosclerosis, and diabetes, which are all diseases that have been associated with reduced life expectancy and premature death.

This category also includes chronic inflammation, including high levels of the proinflammatory markers interleukin-6, tumor necrosis factor, and C-reactive protein. All these markers are also clearly recognized predictors of reduced life expectancy.

Specific diseases

The most important disease in this category is cancer. Cancer has a profound impact on life expectancy, particularly once it has progressed to metastatic disease. The outcomes of this group of diseases are frequently more homogeneous and thus easier to prognosticate. Significant research has revealed the natural course of different types of cancer, including prognosis and survival after diagnosis. Another group in this category includes chronic diseases associated with the failure of vital organs (*e.g.*, congestive heart failure, chronic obstructive pulmonary disease, cirrhosis of the liver, chronic renal insufficiency, and dementia). While these diseases all lead to compromised physiological strength, the outcomes are less homogeneous and predictable than those associated with cancer. Thus, determining the life expectancy of these patients can be more difficult.

The overall increase in the elderly population over the past few years has led to the recognition of a group of symptoms and syndromes that are not yet completely understood. Among these are delirium, malnutrition, cachexia, frailty, and failure to thrive. These syndromes are ominous signs of failure and imminent death. Depression also needs to be included in this group. While depression is not directly fatal by itself (although it can lead to suicide), it amplifies a poor prognosis associated with other pathological processes.

Symptoms

Progressive decreases in food and fluid intake are also reliable markers of a poor prognosis in the elderly. Not eating and drinking is probably *the* most reliable predictor of death of a patient within the two weeks to follow. Anorexia, xerostomia, dysphagia, shortness of breath, and delirium have also been identified as reliable markers of imminent death in cancer patients.

Summary

Specific indicators that are important for the process of prognostication have been reviewed in this chapter. While some of these markers are theoretical, others are clearly more practical. The maximal life span for humans in the current environment is ~100 years. While one's genetic characteristics must be congruent with the environment if one is to reach this advanced age, the same environment will not necessarily produce the same results for all individuals. Likewise, each individual has a distinct potential life span. Any test that measures or that can be used to discover aging or organ dysfunction of any kind may lead to potential markers of reduced life expectancy. Other issues important to patient prognostication were also considered, for example, how one's body typically responds to disease, changes in these responses due to aging, the concept of organ failure, and markers of reduced life expectancy.

In the next chapter, we will address the methods currently used to determine patient prognosis.

CHAPTER 4

Methods Used to Determine Life Expectancy

The most rapidly growing segment of the United States population includes those individuals who are eighty-five years of age and older. Elderly individuals will have reduced physiologic reserves and are thus less likely to recover physiologic homeostasis after a pathophysiologic insult. In this chapter, we review the various tools that can be used to evaluate and determine the prognosis of elderly patients. While each of these tools features several advantages and limitations, collectively they highlight the impact of chronological age, sex, comorbidities, clinical evidence of vital organ damage, a terminal diagnosis, and inability to function and thus maintain homeostasis as predictors of future life expectancy.

Objectives

The goals of this section are

- to review information about mortality;
- to familiarize physicians with life expectancy tables;
- to provide physicians with a general overview of the tools available to determine life expectancy;
- to examine the advantages and limitations of these tools; and
- to identify the factors that are consistently identified as strong predictors of a reduced life expectancy.

Introduction

After reviewing the factors that contribute to human life expectancy in general, the next step is to examine the resources available to determine the life expectancy of an individual patient. The amount of information on this subject is monumental and diverse. Some of these published insights are more useful than others for general clinical practice. In this chapter, we will review examples of available resources that may help a physician tasked with making that determination.

Vital statistics

The median life expectancy for humans has increased significantly over the past one hundred years. As discussed in an earlier chapter, the average human life expectancy, which was 47.3 years in 1900, increased to 77.5 years in 2003.

The increase in life expectancy, together with the population increase (*i.e.*, the baby boom) during the 1950s to early 1960s has changed the profile of the US population. People are living longer (figure 4.1), including those affected by chronic diseases and disabilities.

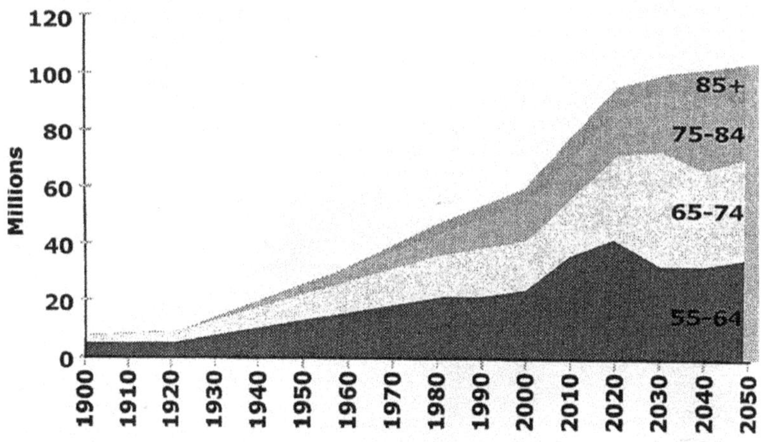

Figure 4.1. Distribution of ages in the US population at years indicated

The most rapidly growing segment of the population includes those eighty-five years of age and older. This is also the group with the least physiological strength. The findings shown earlier in figure 2.3 represent the functional abilities of the elderly population divided by specific age groups. As shown, these individuals become increasingly frail and dependent as they age.

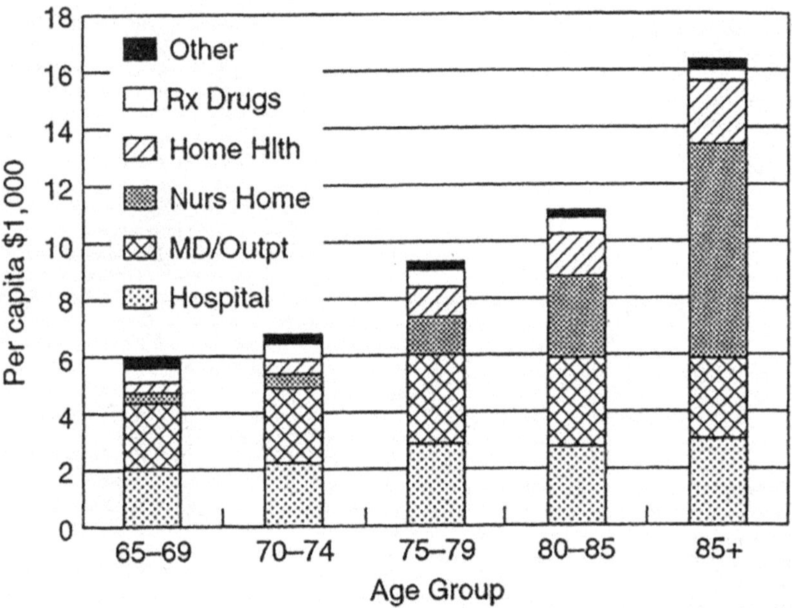

Figure 4.2. Per capita costs of health care in the United States by age

As individuals age, their medical care becomes increasingly expensive. As shown in figure 4.2, elderly individuals use more health care resources than any other group. Most findings suggest that most health care expenditures in the US are for those individuals who are in their final year, final month, and final week of life. In other words, significant resources are used to prevent unavoidable *natural death*.

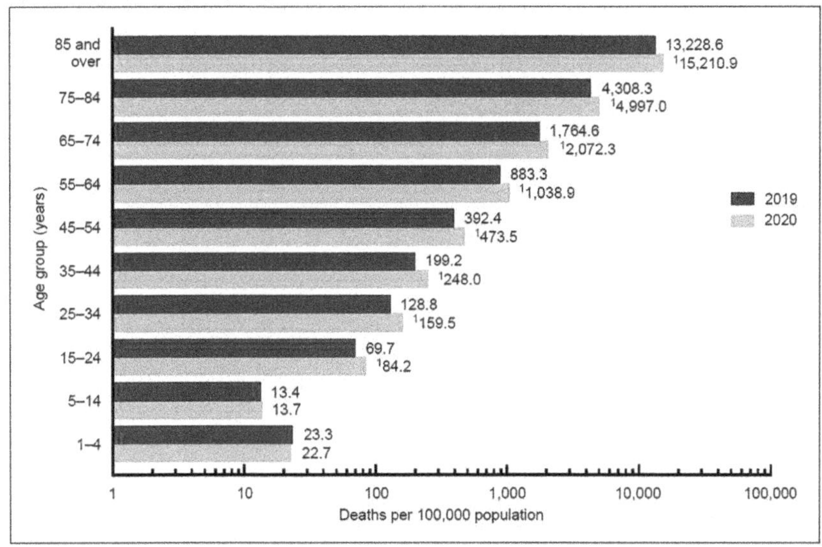

Figure 4.3. Death rates for ages one year and over: US, 2019 and 2020[20]

[1]Statistically significant increase in age-specific death rate from 2019 to 2020 ($p < .05$).

Notes: Rates are plotted on a logarithmic scale. The data table for figure 4.3 includes the number of deaths. Access data table for figure 4.3 at https://www.cdc.gov/nchs/data/databriefs/db427-tables.pdf#3.

Source: National Center for Health Statistics, National Vital Statistics System, Mortality.

Per census data, over three million people died during the year 2020.[21] The death rate begins to increase at age forty-five and increases at a more rapid rate after age sixty-five. In absolute numbers, more than half the deaths were recorded in persons older than seventy-five and three-quarters in people older than sixty-five years of age.

---

[20] NCHS Data Brief, No. 427, December 2021, "Mortality in the United States, 2020," by Sherry L. Murphy, BS, et al., available at https://www.cdc.gov/nchs/data/databriefs/db427.pdf.

[21] Data available at https://www.census.gov/library/stories/2022/03/united-states-deaths-spiked-as-covid-19-continued.html.

Figure 4. Age-adjusted death rates for the 10 leading causes of death in 2020: United States, 2019 and 2020

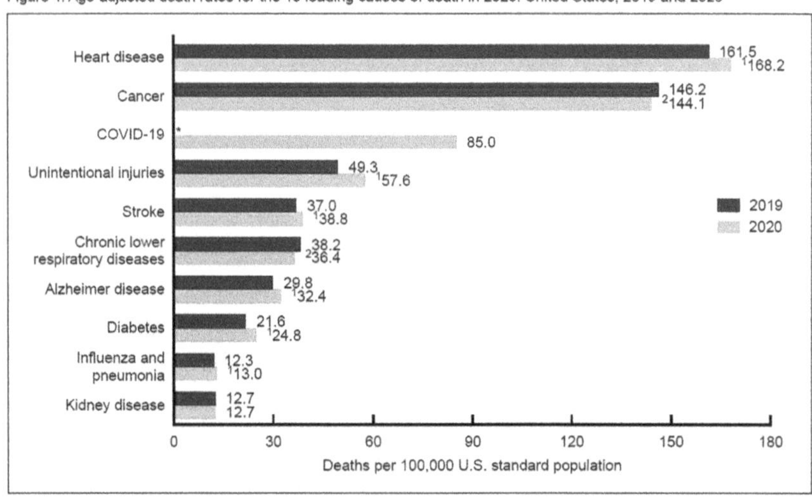

Figure 4.4. Age-adjusted death rates for the ten leading causes of death in 2020: US, 2019 and 2020[22]

*COVID-19 became an official cause of death in 2020; rates for 2019 are not applicable.

[1]Statistically significant increase in age-adjusted death rate from 2019 to 2020 ($p < .05$).

[2]Statistically significant decrease in age-adjusted death rate from 2019 to 2020 ($p < .05$).

Notes: A total of 3,383,729 resident deaths were registered in the United States in 2020. The ten leading causes of death accounted for 74.1% of all deaths in the United States in 2020. Causes of death are ranked according to the number of deaths. Rankings for 2019 data are not shown. Data table for figure 4.4 includes the number of deaths for leading causes and the percentage of total deaths. Access data table for figure 4.4 at https://www.cdc.gov/nchs/data/databriefs/db427-tables.pdf#4.

Source: National Center for Health Statistics, National Vital Statistics System, Mortality.

---

[22] NCHS Data Brief, No. 427, December 2021, "Mortality in the United States, 2020," by Sherry L. Murphy, BS, et al., available at https://www.cdc.gov/nchs/data/databriefs/db427.pdf.

Most of the individuals in this population died from chronic diseases, primarily ischemic heart disease, followed by cancer, stroke, and chronic lower respiratory tract disorders (figure 4.4). The leading cause of death changes over time. In the last two years, the COVID-19 epidemic altered leading causes of death and shortened the overall life expectancy. It is important to note that deaths attributed to chronic respiratory disease and Alzheimer's disease are increasing. This information provides physicians with a framework focused on some of the more critical issues that they will encounter. Appropriate use of this knowledge will enable them to predict how much longer a specific patient is likely to live.

Life expectancy tables

The issue of life expectancy has been analyzed from different perspectives and by different disciplines. While their approach and underlying motivations differ from those of physicians, life insurance companies have expended the most time and effort in the attempt to quantify these issues. Life insurance companies are interested in identifying individuals who are unlikely to die prematurely while they are insured. To select the ideal individuals, they evaluate the same data that we have discussed so far, including family history, age, sex, and body mass index. They also evaluate habits and risk-taking behavior, dangerous pursuits (e.g., racing cars and flying planes), tobacco use, illicit drugs, and type of job. As part of their medical evaluations, insurance companies consider the effects of excessive stress, largely based on diagnoses that include hypertension, metabolic syndrome, abnormal lipid profile, and markers of chronic inflammation. Any individual with evidence of organ damage becomes uninsurable or is faced with a very high premium for very limited coverage. The information on life expectancy shown in table 4.3 explains why most of the life insurance coverage ends at age sixty-five.

Unfortunately, the life expectancy tables developed by life insurance companies are not for public use. These tables might be an excellent tool used in a physician's office. They might be used to motivate patients to address some of their modifiable risk factors and to follow them over time. However, similar to the issues associated with mortality tables, insurance tables will not provide a physician with insight into the life expectancy of an individual patient.

Table 4.1. Provisional expectation of life, by age, Hispanic origin, race for the non-Hispanic population, and sex: United States, 2020. Vital Statistics Surveillance Report

Age (years)	All races and origins			Hispanic			Non-Hispanic white			Non-Hispanic black		
	Total	Male	Female	Total	Male	Female	Total	Male	Female	Total	Male	Female
0	77.3	74.5	80.2	78.8	75.3	82.4	77.6	75.0	80.2	71.8	68.0	75.7
1	76.7	73.9	79.6	78.2	74.7	81.8	76.9	74.3	79.5	71.6	67.8	75.4
5	72.8	70.0	75.6	74.2	70.8	77.8	73.0	70.4	75.6	67.7	63.9	71.5
10	67.8	65.0	70.7	69.3	65.8	72.8	68.0	65.5	70.6	62.8	59.0	66.6
15	62.9	60.1	65.7	64.3	60.9	67.9	63.0	60.5	65.6	57.9	54.1	61.7
20	58.0	55.3	60.8	59.5	56.1	63.0	58.2	55.7	60.7	53.2	49.6	56.8
25	53.3	50.8	56.0	54.7	51.5	58.1	53.4	51.1	55.9	48.8	45.3	52.1
30	48.7	46.2	51.2	50.1	46.9	53.3	48.8	46.5	51.1	44.3	41.0	47.4
35	44.1	41.8	46.5	45.4	42.4	48.5	44.2	42.1	46.4	39.9	36.8	42.8
40	39.6	37.4	41.8	40.8	37.9	43.7	39.7	37.6	41.7	35.6	32.6	38.3
45	35.1	33.0	37.2	36.2	33.5	39.0	35.2	33.3	37.1	31.3	28.6	33.9
50	30.7	28.7	32.7	31.8	29.2	34.4	30.8	29.0	32.6	27.3	24.6	29.6
55	26.5	24.7	28.3	27.6	25.1	29.9	26.6	24.9	28.2	23.4	21.0	25.6
60	22.6	20.9	24.1	23.6	21.3	25.7	22.6	21.1	24.0	19.8	17.6	21.7
65	18.8	17.4	20.1	19.8	17.8	21.6	18.8	17.5	20.0	16.6	14.7	18.2
70	15.3	14.1	16.3	16.4	14.7	17.8	15.2	14.1	16.1	13.7	12.1	15.0
75	12.0	11.1	12.8	13.2	11.8	14.2	11.8	10.9	12.5	11.1	9.8	11.9
80	9.1	8.4	9.6	10.4	9.3	11.1	8.8	8.2	9.3	8.7	7.8	9.3
85	6.7	6.2	7.0	8.1	7.3	8.6	6.4	5.9	6.6	6.7	6.1	7.0

Notes: Life tables by Hispanic origin are based on death rates that have been adjusted for race and ethnicity misclassification on death certificates. Updated classification ratios were applied; see Technical Notes: Estimates are based on provisional data for 2020. Provisional data are subject to change as additional data are received.

Source: National Center for Health Statistics, National Vital Statistics System, Mortality, 2020.

Other life expectancy tables are published and updated periodically, such as the one shown in table 4.1. These tables may provide physicians with useful information that can be used at the bedside and in the office. If a physician has some insight into the years of life expectancy for a given age group, the possible benefits of the therapies offered to the patient will be more clearly understood.

According to the information presented in table 4.1, individuals who have reached eighty-five years of age have an average life expectancy of about seven years. Some of the therapies recommended for the treatment of chronic disease, for example, strict control of hypertension, diabetes, and serum lipid levels, need to be administered for at least seven years to show effectiveness. The same scenario applies to screening measures. Most evidence suggests these screenings provide little to no benefit for those with an average life expectancy of less than 5–10 years. It is important to note that an individual who is one hundred years old has on average only 2.6 more years of life expectancy; these findings are in agreement with what we have reviewed previously.[23]

Considering that the maximal life expectancy has not changed, it will be critical to question the benefit of many of these recommendations. It is still not clear whether elderly individuals might stay functional for longer periods by following these recommendations and, by doing so, decrease the likelihood of prolonged illness, dependence, and excessive medical costs.

---

[23] Data derived from National Vital Statistics Report, Volume 54, Number 14, "United States Life Tables, 2003, revised as of March 28, 2007," Table A, indicating life expectancy at one hundred years of age is overall 2.5 years. Available at https://www.cdc.gov/nchs/data/nvsr/nvsr54/nvsr54_14.pdf.

Tools used to determine life expectancy

Several instruments have been developed that provide more accurate predictions of the life expectancy of an individual patient. Most of these tools have been created by performing complex statistical analyses of characteristics unique to the patients who die among those followed over a specific period. The tools typically introduce a scoring system that focuses on the statistically significant characteristics among members of this specific cohort. The risk of dying within a given period is usually expressed by a percentage, with higher values assigned to patients at greater risk.

There is currently a large number and variety of tools that can be used to prognosticate patients. These tools are classified below (table 4.4) based on their common characteristics, including settings, type of medical issue addressed, and time periods.

Table 4.2. Tools for patient prognostication

Settings	Medical issues		Time periods
Emergency department	Brain injury	Cancer	Mortality during the index admission
	Trauma	Pneumonia	
Intensive care unit			Mortality after the index admission
	Presurgical evaluation	Chronic obstructive pulmonary disease	
In-hospital			From three months to several years
Outpatient	Myocardial infarction	Cerebrovascular accident	
Nursing home			
	Congestive heart failure	Palliative care	
		Hospice	

These tools each have unique predictive values. While a review of all tools that might be used in this situation is beyond the scope of this book, the remaining sections of this chapter will focus on representative tools designed for use in inpatient and outpatient settings, as well as palliative care and hospice.

Examples

The first example relates to a physician's capacity to predict death (table 4.3).

Table 4.3. Physician-based assessment of the severity of illness

Severity	Not ill	Mildly	Moderately	Severely	Moribund
Score	1	2–3	4–5	6–7	8–9
Mortality (%)	0	0–2	3–6	21–24	55–62

Reprinted from M. E. Charlson et al., "Assessing Illness Severity," J. Chronic Disease 39, no. 6 (1986): 439–452.

In 1986, M. E. Charlson published findings that focused on the accuracy of physicians-in-training when asked to predict when an individual patient might be expected to die based on the severity of the illness at admission measured on a scale from 0 (not ill) to 9 (moribund). The physicians-in-training were fairly accurate in predicting death and most accurate when the patient was classified as moribund.

The *Glasgow Coma Scale* is another measurement used routinely in hospital practice. This scale is used by emergency physicians to determine the neurological status of patients presenting with brain injury. This instrument is fairly accurate not only in determining the severity of the brain injury but also the risk of imminent death. Similarly the Apache II score used in an intensive care setting to predict the outcomes of acute diseases is also an excellent predictor of patient survival.

The next example focuses on the risk of dying when the patient is admitted to the hospital for pneumonia.

Table 4.4. Burden of Illness Scores for Elderly Persons (BISEP). (Inoye, Sharon, K. Page, et al., "Medical Care," *Bi Sep* 41, no. 1 [2003]: 17–83.)

Relative risk	Score	Relative risk	Score
Lymphoma/leukemia	6	Chronic lung disease	2
Acute renal insufficiency	5	Chronic renal insufficiency	2
Metastatic cancer	3	DM with end organ damage	1
Localized cancer	3	Pneumonia	1
CVA	2		
CHF	2		
Total score			

Relative risk group	Score	Final points
Group A	0	0
Group B	1–2	1
Group C	3–5	2
Group D	≥6	3

Item	Score	Points
Relative risk final points	Max. of 6	-
Albumin	≤3.5	1
Serum creatinine	≥1.5	1
Dementia before admission	+	1
Function	Needing help to walk or not able to do it	1
Total points		

Total points	0 1	2	3	4 5 6 7
Group	1	II	III	IV
Mortality at one year (%)	5–8	17–24	33–51	61–74

Reprinted from Inouye S. K. et al., Med Care 2003; 41(1) 70–83.

Pneumonia is among the most frequent diagnoses leading to death in hospitalized chronically ill and frail elderly patients. The Burden of Illness Score for Elderly Persons (BISEP; table 4.6) focuses on the extent of chronic disease together with markers of organ damage, for example, low albumin and high creatinine levels. This tool highlights the significance of dementia and overall function when generating a specific patient score.

Another instrument that is commonly used to measure the risk of dying during a surgical procedure is the Modified Cardiac Risk Index (figure 4.5).

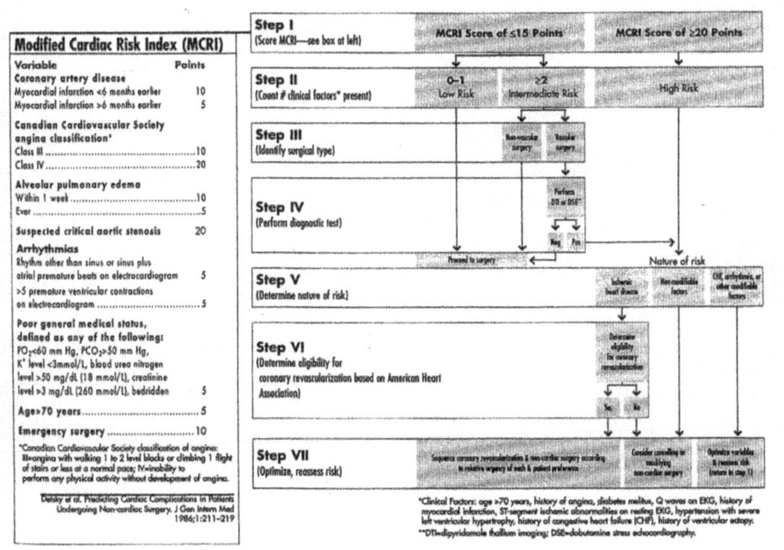

Figure 4.5. Modified Cardiac Risk Index (MCRI). *Reprinted from Detsky AS et al. J Gen Internal Med 1986; 1(4): 211–219.*

As part of this tool, which focuses on a value known as the Modified Cardiac Risk Index, any patient who scores twenty or more points is identified as part of the "high-risk" group and is generally in poor condition. This tool provides significant weight when considering age, function, and evidence of vital organ damage. While this tool is not designed to assess survival, patients identified as unlikely to be able to tolerate a surgical procedure are also those at risk of dying as a result of the condition that brought him/her to the hospital.

Other forms and scoring systems have been designed for use in outpatient settings. Among these is the "Four-Year Mortality Prognostic Index," which focuses on the mortality risk of patients in the general community (figure 4.6).

Box. Four-Year Mortality Index for Older Adults

1. Age _______________________________   60-64: 1 point
   65-69: 2 points
   70-74: 3 points
   75-79: 4 points
   80-84: 5 points
   ≥85: 7 points

2. Sex (Male/Female)   Male: 2 points

3. a. Weight ____________________   BMI <25: 1 point
   b. Height ____________________

   703 × (weight in pounds/ height in inches)²
   BMI = ____________________

4. Has a doctor ever toldyou that you have diabetes   Diabetes: 2 points
   or high blood sugar? (Y/N)

5. Has a doctor told you that you have cancer or a   Cancer: 2 points
   malignant tumor, excluding minor skin cancers? (Y/N)

6. Do you have a chronic lung disease   Lung Disease: 2 points
   that limits your usual activities or makes
   you need oxygen at home? (Y/N)

7. Has a doctor told you that you have   Heart Failure: 2 points
   congestive heart failure? (Y/N)

8. Have you smoked cigarettes in the past week? (Y/N)   Smoke: 2 points

9. Because of a health or memory problem   Bathing: 2 points
   do you have any difficulty with bathing
   or showering? (Y/N)

10. Because of a health or memory problem,   Finances: 2 points
    do you have any difficulty with managing
    your money—such as paying your bills
    and keeping track of expenses? (Y/N)

11. Because of a health problem do you have   Walking: 2 points
    any difficulty with walking several blocks? (Y/N)

12. Because of a health problem do you have   Push or Pull: 1 point
    any difficulty with pulling or pushing
    large objects like a living room chair? (Y/N)

Total Points: ____________________

Points	4-Year Mortality Risk
0 – 5	3 %
6 – 9	15 %
10 – 13	40 %
≥ 14	67 %

Reference: Spi J Lee, MD; JAMA; February 15, 2006, Vol. 295, No. 7

Figure 4.6. Four-Year Mortality Index for Older Adults.
Reprinted from Lee SJ, JAMA 2006; 295(7); 801–808

Similar to the tools used to evaluate inpatients, this method identifies age, chronic disease load, vital organ damage, and decreased function as significant markers that can be used to identify patients with a reduced life expectancy. It is interesting to note that this scoring system uses advanced age as one of the more significant items for predicting death, particularly if we consider the fact that the subjects under evaluation must be at least somewhat functional as they can still receive care at a physician's office.

Elderly individuals also die while receiving care in nursing homes. Significant interest has developed over the past few years in having a system that would help to identify nursing home patients who are about to die. The purpose of this effort would be to improve the care of these patients by offering them palliative care and hospice services and thus avoiding useless medications or harmful tests and procedures.

The Minimum Dataset (MDS) is a detailed assessment tool created by the Centers for Medicare and Medicaid Services to evaluate, follow, and determine the needs of patients residing in nursing homes. All patients are evaluated at admission and periodically thereafter. They are also evaluated when there is a significant change in their clinical status.

Table 4.5. Minimum Dataset (MDS) from Centers for Medicare and Medicaid Services

MDS items	Assessments with item present	Followed by death within six months
Cognitive measures		
Disorganized speech, recent onset	301	93 (31%)
Periods of lethargy, recent onset	544	212 (39%)
Indicators of depression or anxiety		
Withdrawal from activity daily	884	263 (30%)
ADL and functional ability measures		
Surface transfer did not occur	878	334 (38%)
Walking on unit did not occur	2,655	851 (32%)

Dressing did not occur	295	113 (38%)
Eating did not occur	149	66 (44%)
Did not use toilet	442	132 (30%)
Did not get out of bed	3,326	1,047 (31%)
Health conditions and problems		
Dehydration	188	85 (45%)
Insufficient fluid intake[a]	563	261 (46%)
Recurrent lung aspirations[a]	566	199 (35%)
Terminal diagnosis	1,573	751 (48%)
Nutritional/oral/dental status		
Parenteral/IV	758	243 (32%)
Oral debris[a]	44	16 (36%)
Skin ulcers		
Five or more skin ulcers	1,008	336 (33%)
Time awake and activity involvement		
Not awake in morning, afternoon, or evening	1,286	400 (31%)
Involved in activities less than one-third of time	4,218	1,258 (30%)
Never involved in activities	202	68 (34%)
Prefers change in types of activities[a]	51	23 (45%)
Prefers change in involvement level[a]	67	27 (40%)
Special treatments and procedures		
Receives suctioning[a]	612	199 (33%)

[a]Items included in only full MDS assessments

Table 4.6. Death rates associated with the MDS. Assessments with multiple items present after which the resident died within six months

Number of items present	n	Followed by death within six months
One or more	12,256	3,318 (27.1%)
Two or more	4,360	1,651 (37.9%)

Three or more	2,059	918 (44.6%)
Four or more	1,037	530 (51.1%)
Five or more	526	308 (58.6%)
Six or more	219	147 (67.1%)
Seven or more	97	66 (68.0%)
Eight or more	38	25 (65.8%)
Nine or more	10	7 (70.0%)
Ten or more	5	4 (80.0%)

The information presented in table 4.7 highlights the items included in the MDS that show statistically significant differences in patients who die within the six months to follow. Table 4.8 lists the probability of death according to the number of these significant characteristics identified in a given patient. As shown, the inability to maintain hydration and nutrition, followed by decreases in motivation and function as measured by ADLs, is a significant marker indicating the likelihood of patient demise within the following six months.

Several tools have been created to determine whether a patient is a candidate for palliative care or hospice. These tools are very helpful at the bedside and can be used to identify patients with very short life expectancy. The form shown in figure 4.6 is an example of a tool used by the Palliative Center in Lexington, Kentucky, to determine patient eligibility for their services.

Table 4.7. Palliative Care Screening Tool. Source: Adapted from Palliative Care Center of the Bluegrass, Lexington, KY

Criteria—please consider the following criteria when determining the palliative care score of this patient	
1. Basic disease process	Scoring
a. Cancer (metastatic/recurrent)	Score 2 points each
b. Advanced COPD	
c. Stroke (with decreased function by at least 50%)	
d. End-stage renal disease	
e. Advanced cardiac disease—i.e., CHF, severe CAD, CM (LVEF < 25%)	
f. Other life-limiting illness	

2. Concomitant disease processes
  a. Liver disease
  b. Moderate renal disease
  c. Moderate COPD
  d. Moderate congestive heart failure
  e. Other condition complicating care
	Score 1 point overall

3. Functional status of patient Using ECOG Performance Status (Eastern Cooperative Oncology Group)	Score as specified below

ECOG	Grade	Scale	
	0	Fully active, able to carry on all predisease activities without restriction	Score 0
	1	Restricted in physically strenuous activity but ambulatory and able to carry out work of a light or sedentary nature, e.g., light housework, office work	Score 0
	2	Ambulatory and capable of all self-care but unable to carry out any work activities, up and about more than 50% of waking hours	Score 1
	3	Capable of only limited self-care; confined to bed or chair more than 50% of waking hours	Score 2
	4	Completely disabled, cannot carry on any self-care, totally confined to bed or chair	Score 3

4. Other criteria to consider in screening	Score 1 pt. each
• Team/patient/family needs help with complex decision-making and determination of goals of care	_____________
• Patient has unacceptable level of pain or other symptom distress > 24 hours	_____________
• Patient has uncontrolled psychosocial or spiritual issues	_____________

PROGNOSTICATION

- Patient has frequent visits to emergency department (>1× mo for same diagnosis)   _________

- Patient has more than one hospital admission for
  the same diagnosis in last 30 days   _________

- Patient has prolonged length of stay (>five days)
  without evidence of progress   _________

- Patient has prolonged stay in ICU and/or trans-
  ferred from ICU to ICU setting without evidence
  of progress   _________

- Patient is in an ICU setting with documented
  poor prognosis   _________

Total score	_________

Scoring guidelines	Total score = 2 no intervention needed
	Total score = 3 observation only
	Total score = 4 consider palliative care consult (requires physician order)

_________________________________   _____________________

Signature of staff member completing form   Date

PALLIATIVE CARE SCREENING TOOL

Source: Adapted from Palliative Care Center of the Bluegrass, Lexington, Kentucky

Criteria—Please consider the following criteria when determining the palliative care score of this patient	
1. Basic disease process a. Cancer (Metastatic/Recurrent) d. End stage renal disease b. Advanced COPD e. Advanced cardiac disease—i.e., CHF, severe CAD, CM (LVEF<25%) c. Stroke (with decreased function by at least 50%) f. Other life-limiting illness	SCORING SCORE 2 POINTS EACH
2. Concomitant disease processes a. Liver disease d. Moderate congestive heart failure b. Moderate renal disease e. Other condition complicating care c. Moderate COPD	SCORE 1 POINT OVERALL
3. Functional status of patient Using ECOG Performance Status (Eastern Cooperative Oncology Group)	SCORE AS SPECIFIED BELOW

ECOG	Grade	Scale	
	0	Fully Active, able to carry on all pre-disease activities without restriction	SCORE 0
	1	Restricted in physically strenuous activity but ambulatory and able to carry out work of a light or sedentary nature, e.g., light housework, office work	SCORE 0
	2	Ambulatory and capable of all self-care but unable to carry out any work activities, up and about more than 50% of waking hours	SCORE 1
	3	Capable of only limited self-care; confined to bed or chair more than 50% of waking hours	SCORE 2
	4	Completely disabled, cannot carry on any self-care, totally confined to bed or chair	SCORE 3

4. Other criteria to consider in screening	SCORE 1 PT EACH
• Team/patient/family needs help with complex decision-making and determination of goals of care	
• Patient has unacceptable level of pain or other symptom distress > 24 hours	
• Patient has uncontrolled psychosocial or spiritual issues	
• Patient has frequent visits to emergency department (>1 x mo for same diagnosis)	
• Patient has more than one hospital admission for the same diagnosis in last 30 days	
• Patient has prolonged length of stay (> five days) without evidence of progress	
• Patient has prolonged stay in ICU and/or transferred from ICU to ICU setting without evidence of progress	
• Patient is in an ICU setting with documented poor prognosis	
TOTAL SCORE	

SCORING GUIDELINES:
TOTAL SCORE = 2 No intervention needed
TOTAL SCORE = 3 Observation only
TOTAL SCORE = 4 Consider Palliative Care Consult (requires physician order)

____   __________

Signature of Staff Member Completing Form   Date

Figure 4.7. Palliative Care Screening Tool. Adapted from Palliative Care Center of the Bluegrass, Paducah, Kentucky, US.

The Palliative Care Screening Tool focuses on the diagnosis of a terminal disease, chronic disease load, and functional impairment as determining factors. Other markers of poor prognosis featured in this tool include frequent visits to the emergency department, recent admissions to the hospital for the same problem, the length of stay in the hospital and the intensive care unit, and the need for help in decision-making and/or conflict resolution.

Hospice care facilities have developed disease-specific criteria to determine if a patient is a candidate to receive their services. The criteria are based primarily on our current understanding of the natural course of the disease (table 4.9).

Table 4.8. Criteria for consideration of a palliative care consultation

Condition	Criteria
Heart disease	Symptoms of CHF at rest Ejection fraction < 20% New dysrhythmia Cardiac arrest, syncope, or CVA Frequent emergency room visits for symptoms
Cancer	All metastatic or inoperable disease
Pulmonary disease	Dyspnea at rest Signs or symptoms of right heart failure Hypoxemia (with administration of oxygen) FEV1 < 30% $pCO_2 > 50$ Unintentional weight loss (>10% of body weight)
Cerebrovascular accident	Acute phase unchanged, beyond 3 days Coma Absent verbal response Absent withdrawal to pain Kamofsky score, <50% Recurrent aspiration pneumonia Dysphagia precluding nutrition

Dementia	Inability to walk Incontinence Fewer than 6 meaningful words Albumin <2.5 g/dL or decreased oral intake Nutritional compromise Severe medical comorbidities Frequent emergency room visits
Liver disease	Not considered candidate for transplant Prothrombin time >5 seconds over control Albumin <2.5 g/dL Refractory ascites Spontaneous bacterial peritonitis Jaundice Malnutrition and muscle wasting
Renal disease	Not a candidate for dialysis Creatinine clearance <15 mL/min Serum creatinine level >8.0 mg/dL (6.0 mg/dL if diabetic)
Amyotrophic lateral sclerosis	Dysphagia requiring a feeding tube Dyspnea or symptoms of hypoventilation; forced vital capacity of 50% or less Loss of function in two body regions (bulbar, arms or legs) Pain requiring high doses of analgesic medications Severe psychological and/or social or spiritual distress or suffering
Failure to thrive	Frequent emergency room visits Albumin <2.5 g/dL Unintentional weight loss Decubitus ulcers Homebound/bed confined

This table is a simplified version of the criteria used by a hospice to determine patient eligibility for their services. The use of these criteria at the bedside helps determine not only the patient's prognosis but also services that may be needed after discharge from the hospital.

The Medicare requirements for hospice services also include function as a significant part of the evaluation. Table 4.10 outlines the scale used by Medicare services to measure patient function.

Table 4.9. The Palliative Performance Scale (PPS)

%	Ambulation	Activity and evidence of disease	Self-care	Intake	Level of consciousness
100	Full	Normal activity, no evidence of disease	Full	Normal	Full
90	Full	Normal activity, some evidence of disease	Full	Normal	Full
80	Full	Normal activity with effort, some evidence of disease	Full	Normal or reduced	Full
70	Reduced	Unable to do normal work, some evidence of disease	Full	Normal or reduced	Full
60	Reduced	Unable to do hobby or some housework, significant disease	Occasional assistance	Normal or reduced	Full or confusion
50	Mainly sit/lie	Unable to do any work, extensive disease	Considerable assistance	Normal or reduced	Full or confusion
40	Mainly in bed	Unable to do any work, extensive disease	Mainly assistance	Normal or reduced	Any

30	Totally bedbound	Unable to do any work, extensive disease	Total care	Reduced	Any
20	Totally bedbound	Unable to do any work, extensive disease	Total care	Minimal sips	Any
10	Totally bedbound	Unable to do any work, extensive disease	Total care	Mouth care only	Drowsy or coma
0	Death	-	-	-	-

The Palliative Performance Scale (PPS) is a strong and consistent predictor of imminent death and is particularly useful in patients with a functional capacity of 30 percent or lower. As shown, the lower the score, the worse the prognosis.

The group of signs and symptoms that comprise the Syndrome of Imminent Death is probably the most reliable predictor of this condition. Patients who enter this trajectory typically live fourteen days or fewer thereafter (table 4.11).

Table 4.10. Stages of the Syndrome of Imminent Death

1. *Stages*

   Early

   - Bedbound
   - Loss of interest and/or ability to drink/eat
   - Cognitive changes: increasing time spent sleeping and/or delirium (see Fast Fact #1).

   Mid

   - Further decline in mental status to obtundation (slow to arouse with stimulation; only brief periods of wakefulness)

- Death rattle—pooled oral sections that are not cleared due to loss of swallowing reflex

Late

- Coma
- Fever: usually from aspiration pneumonia
- Altered respiratory pattern—periods of apnea, hyperpnea, or irregular breathing
- Mottled extremities

2. *Time course.* The time to traverse the various stages can be less than twenty-four hours or as long as fourteen days. Patients who enter the trajectory who are nutritionally intact, with no infection (e.g., acute stroke), are apt to live longer than cachectic cancer patients.

Reprinted from D. E. Weissman, "Syndrome of Imminent Death," *Fast Fact and Concept* 3, 2nd ed. (July 2005), End-of-Life-Palliative Care Network of Wisconsin, https://www.mypcnow.org/fast-fact/syndrome-of-imminent-death/.

Advantages of these tools

When the tools are used in the setting for which they were designed, they can provide the physician with a general idea of the prognosis of each patient at a given moment in time. The use of an appropriate form for each setting might provide the physician with insight into the decline of the patient as they transition from the office to the hospital (in situations of acute events) or nursing home and forward through the last moments of life. These tools are indirect measures of a patient's physiological reserves and can be used to adjust therapies provided based on his or her anticipated life expectancy. The instruments used by palliative care and hospice help to determine the severity of the disease and the appropriate place of discharge and services needed.

Limitations of the tools

These tools were developed based on statistically significant characteristics identified in patients with very short life expectancies that were adjusted for the nature of a given population, medical issues, and the lengths of time that were studied. It is important to note that these are only snapshots of the dying process experienced by individual patients. These tools do not consider other important information that may contribute to patient prognosis. This is probably why even the best and most experienced prognosticators cannot accurately predict the time of death more than 70 percent of the time. At the bedside, these instruments cannot provide the physician with specific insight into whether a particular patient might be assigned to the group that is going to live or the group that is going to die.

Prognosticating instruments do not consider the severity of the insult or the response (or lack of response) to treatment, which are of course all important factors that determine the potential survival of an individual patient. In reality, it is impractical to have to use different tools for different types of situations. However, even with their limitations, these tools can still be helpful when used to estimate overall patient prognosis.

Markers of a reduced life expectancy

No matter how complicated the data and the statistical analysis, most tools consistently identify and focus on a single set of markers as the best predictors of a reduced life expectancy. These markers include older age, male sex, severity of the observed decrease in function, chronic disease load or comorbidities, evidence of vital organ damage, carrying a terminal diagnosis, and inability to maintain homeostasis.

Summary

In this chapter, we reviewed useful information and resources that are readily available that can be used by physicians to identify patients with poor prognoses at different levels of care. We also examined the advantages and disadvantages of these tools. Most importantly, a set of markers that can be used in the process of prognostication were identified.

In the next chapter, we will discuss the mental process that might be followed by clinicians who are tasked with determining the prognosis of an individual patient.

CHAPTER 5

Process

In this chapter, we will use the information discussed earlier in the text to generate a framework to determine the prognosis of an individual patient. Here we introduce a four-step structured process that begins with an assessment of the patient's baseline state, an initial characterization of the disease manifestations, and the patient's response to treatment. Based on these findings, an individualized patient prognosis can then be generated. We recognize that the results of prognostication are inexact and that many potential surprises and "gray" zones can emerge along the way. However, this method provides a structured format for physicians who are attempting to identify the most humane and appropriate strategies and objectives for managing the care of their elderly patients.

Objectives

The goals of this section are as follows:

- To lay out the framework for the process of prognostication
- To review the factors that identify the position of a specific patient on the curve of decline and the process used to determine the prognosis of an individual patient

Introduction

Following the information provided in previous chapters, we will now assemble the important pieces so that we can understand the process of prognostication. The first chapter in this book provided us with a general idea of the importance of this process, notably those factors that focus on physician perceptions and the benefits associated with the process of prognostication. In the second chapter, we reviewed concepts that are important to the understanding of the process, including senescence, aging, and the significance of organ failure. In chapter 3, we reviewed the factors that limit potential life expectancy. In chapter 4, we went one step further and reviewed statistically significant characteristics identified in the literature that are present in patients with reduced life expectancies. In this chapter, we will continue to review these factors and consolidate them in an easy, practical, and comprehensible way to facilitate our understanding of their role in the process used to determine patient prognosis.

Factors that determine patient prognosis

As discussed in previous chapters, and from a practical point of view, a patient's ability to maintain a viable microenvironment will be largely dependent on the physiological strength available that can be used to compensate for the imbalance resulting from a disease process or trauma (table 5.1).

Table 5.1. Factors that determine prognosis

Physiological strength	Disease process
Age	Speed of the attack
Function	Intensity
Chronic disease load	Duration
Vital organ failure—number and severity	Extent and severity of the damage
Presence of malnutrition, delirium, dementia, and depression	Organs affected

Physiological strength

There are no simple or practical ways to measure an individual's physiological strength. However, one can make an educated guess by considering the factors identified in the previous chapter (chronological age, male sex, and others) that consistently predicted patient demise.

Collectively, these factors can provide the physician with a "snapshot" of where the patient is on his or her personal trajectory of decline. The first three factors determine how a patient compares with similar populations, reflected by his or her physiological age (figure 5.1). The final four factors determine the strength of the remaining physiological reserves.

Chronological age is the best predictor of death for the healthy elderly population. These individuals exhibit a rate of decline that would be expected in response to normal aging. In this cohort, the physiological and the chronological ages match one another. The situation is quite different for those who have sustained serious illnesses at a younger age and develop vital organ damage. The physiological age of individuals in this cohort will be higher than their chronological age and they are likely to undergo a more rapid decline.

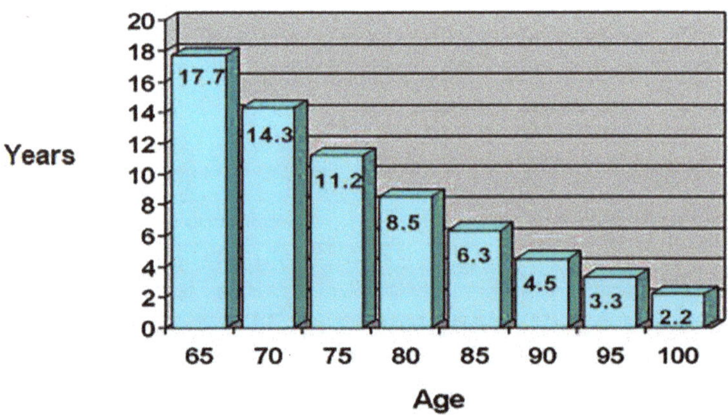

Figure 5.1. Life expectancy in the United States in 1997. Additional years of life expectancy at each age (65–100 years).

The graphic shown in figure 5.1 was created using data from life expectancy tables. This information provides the physician with a general idea of how much longer the cohort of patients in this age group might be expected to live. The significance of these numbers is limited because they present extra years of life for a cohort without differentiating between those who are ill and those who have remained healthy. The graphs shown in figure 5.2 differentiate the population into quartiles based on comorbidities. Based on the third principle (above), patients burdened by significant disease are likely to die sooner.

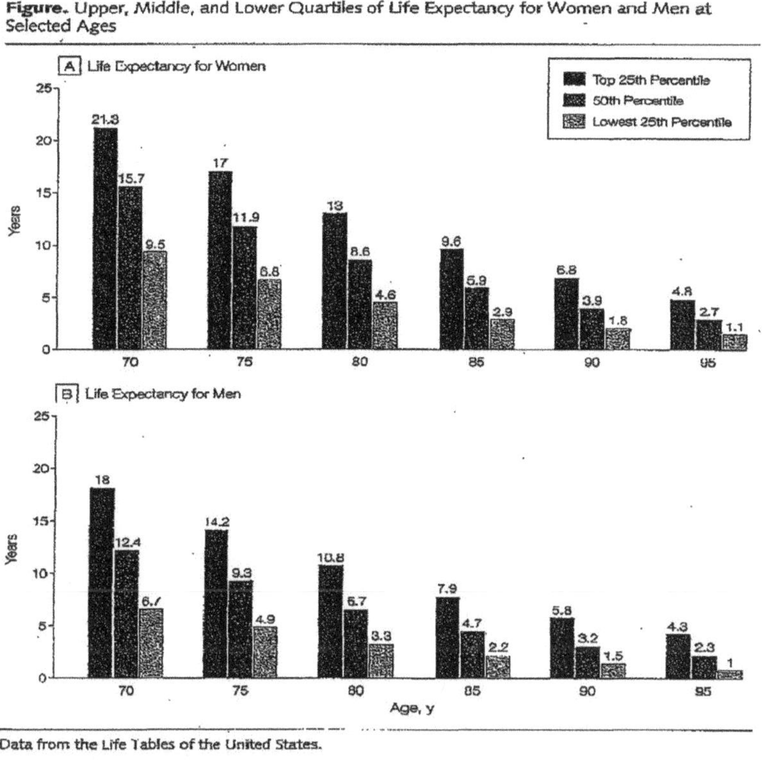

Figure 5.2. Quartiles of life expectancy for men and women aged 70–90 years. *Reprinted from JAMA 285, no. 21 (June 6, 2001).*

Male *versus* female sex is also a factor that determines individual life expectancy. While women live longer than men (figure 5.2), this factor will not add significant value to the process of prognostication when applied to a specific patient.

Function is second only to age among the most important factors determining life expectancy and patient prognosis; this is relevant to all patients, including those who have aged prematurely. Function is a global measure of physiological strength.

All four components of function might need to be evaluated for a full understanding of a decrease in function. It is not unusual to find patients who have a fair cardiovascular reserve but are inactive due to a physical impairment or are demented, delirious, or depressed. Observations that raise these possibilities include the perception of the team that a patient might be capable of doing more, is confused, or consistently answers questions by saying "I don't know." In cases such as these, the use of specific screening tests, such as the Geriatric Depression Scale (GDS) and the Mini-Mental State Evaluation (MMSE), could provide additional insight into these possibilities.

Using these two parameters, i.e., age and function, a physician can compare the patient with the group and determine whether his or her chronological and physiological ages match one another. There are three possible outcomes to this exercise. First, the patient may be strong for his chronological age; this implies that the patient is in the top twenty-fifth percentile. Second, both chronological and physiological ages match one another, implying that the patient would fall in the middle fiftieth percentile. In the third scenario, in which the patient has aged prematurely, he or she will likely be positioned in the lower twenty-fifth percentile and will likely die sooner than the other members of the group.

The next set of markers will provide the physician with more detailed information on the extent to which the patient's ability to maintain homeostasis has been compromised and thus the extent to which his or her life expectancy will be reduced.

Signs and symptoms of organ dysfunction

As discussed in the previous chapter, organ dysfunction ensues when the system has exhausted the normal compensatory mechanisms and is maintaining a reduced level of function. The more severe the damage and the greater the number of organs failing, the less able an individual will be at maintaining homeostasis under situations of stress. It is important to remember that, with respect to immediate survival, the cardiovascular system is most important, followed by the respiratory, metabolic, and renal systems. Renal system failure has become less significant since the development of hemodialysis. With respect to prognostication, dysfunction of the nervous, hematologic, and muscular systems is also significant a marker for a reduced life expectancy.

Malnutrition, delirium, dementia, and depression are all markers of organ dysfunction. The absence of significant reserves can lead to metabolic and central nervous system failure. The contributions of these systems are essential for normal function. Malnutrition could be due to social and/or medical reasons such as lack of personal and/or social resources or being unable to go to the grocery store and prepare meals. Other reasons for this problem may be related to difficulty eating, lack of appetite, or the inability of the body to metabolize food. Regardless of the reason, malnutrition implies failure to thrive. From the prognostication standpoint, medical concerns (i.e., cachexia) are the most significant of these reasons. The inability to maintain hydration and nutrition is also a significant factor and is among the most reliable marker of imminent death. Delirium, dementia, and depression have similar significance for organ failure.

From the practical point of view, we can simplify the factors contributing to the physiological strength of a patient into three specific categories: age, level of function, number, severity of failing and failed organs, and diagnoses of terminal disease.

Severity of the disease process

From the point of view of an insult, survival can only occur if the challenge is sufficiently limited so that the patient's compensatory mechanisms have an opportunity to function and that the response is strong enough to restore homeostasis to an acceptable level (table 5.1). The sufficiency of the compensatory response depends on the patient's baseline reserves and the extent of the damage. The extent of the damage depends on three specific characteristics of the insult:

its speed, intensity, and duration. As a general rule, in a patient with less physiological strength, less organ damage is needed to generate total system failure.

The trauma, occupational medicine, and industry literature includes quite a bit of information on permissible levels of exposure to chemicals, radiation, and the environment, as well as the severity of trauma and resulting symptoms and their treatment. There is currently no practical method for determining the severity of the insults sustained by most patients seen in routine medical practice. However, a physician typically has significant knowledge regarding the natural history of the disease and, of particular note, how the patient might respond to the specific illness. This response is the end result of a complex set of interactions between the nature of the insult and the patient's physiological strength. Of note the patient's initial response is often the best indicator of the severity of an insult.

The process used to determine patient prognosis

The process used to analyze the information and to determine the patient's prognosis is fairly simple. All the information needed for this process is collected as part of the regular practice of medicine. The process includes four basic steps.

Step 1.
<u>BASELINE</u>
Chronological
age
Previous level
of function
Baseline organ
damage

Figure 5.3. The process used to determine prognosis: step 1

The first step is to determine the patient's baseline physiological reserve (figure 5.3). This information can be obtained from the patient's chronological age. As discussed in previous chapters, this value will provide insight into the life expectancy of the patient based on information collected for a cohort of individuals of the same chronological age. Next an assessment of the patient's baseline level of function will permit the physician to determine whether there is a match between the patient's physiological and chronological age. This information will suggest that the patient might be able to live longer, for about the same duration, or shorter than might be expected given his/her chronological age. Baseline markers of vital organ damage as well as the severity of the dysfunction will provide the physician with the information needed to determine the extent to which the patient's physiological strength has been impaired. This is important information needed to estimate the quartile position of each patient shown on the graph in figure 5.2. A patient with more severe vital organ damage will have a reduced life expectancy. Another important element of recent history is the speed of patient decline. A more rapid patient decline will also lead to a reduced life expectancy.

The information collected thus far should be used to modulate the aggressiveness of any treatment or therapies offered to the patient. If the pertinent information is not available, other characteristics, such as whether the patient lives in a nursing home, an assisted living facility, or a dementia unit, history of being bed- or wheelchair-bound at home, and/or detection of contractures and/ or cachexia on physical examination, are all clues that suggest the patient has very low levels of physiological reserve. Also any previous diagnosis including the term "terminal" can be highly significant in this context. Careful use of this step will also help the physician to highlight realistic expectations for the future. As a general rule, except in cases of organ transplants and some corrective surgeries, an elderly patient will not be in better condition after a hospital admission than he or she was before the current index event.

Step 1.
BASELINE
Chronological age
Previous level of function
Baseline organ damage

Step 2. INITIAL ASSESSMENT
Severity of the insult
New organ damage
Reversibility of the damage

Figure 5.4. The process used to determine prognosis: step 2

The second step is to determine the severity of the insult (figure 5.4). This is done by assessing the patient's initial response to the insult. This assessment includes three aspects, all of them equally important and complementary to one another. The first aspect to consider is patient stability. For example, is the patient conscious, confused, pale, cold, sweating, in pain, short of breath, or weak? The second aspect focuses on the vital signs, and the third, on the ability of the patient to maintain the microenvironment (pH, oxygen and carbon dioxide concentrations, and bicarbonate levels, among others). The more these values deviate from the patient's baseline, the poorer the prognosis and the closer the patient is to death. However, it is not unusual in emergency situations to find that the physician will be required to select treatments for a given patient based solely on his or her initial clinical impression.

The initial assessment is not a one-time evaluation. Some insults are episodic, for example, trauma as well as some cerebrovascular accidents or myocardial infarctions. Others develop over a while, for example, kidney infections, pneumonia, or sepsis. A physician might underestimate the severity of the problem if the initial evaluation was performed only at the beginning of the insult. The physician needs to remember that the effects of an initial insult end only when the patient reaches either a point of stability or dies, which may require a substantial amount of time.

The initial assessment, together with the natural history of the disease, will provide the physician with insight into the severity, permanence, or reversibility of the insult. This information will be essential for predicting the patient's survival and future level of function. For example, cases of pneumonia of similar severity will be more detrimental and possibly even lethal in a patient with severe chronic obstructive pulmonary disease than in a normal healthy elderly patient. Similarly different types of cerebrovascular accidents are less well-tolerated in an older person compared to a younger person; this differential is exacerbated in cases in which the patients are demented.

Step 1. **BASELINE**
Chronological age
Previous level of function
Baseline organ damage

Step 2. **INITIAL ASSESSMENT**
Severity of the insult
New organ damage
Reversibility of the damage

Step 3. **RESPONSE TO TREATMENT**
Digression
Stabilization
Improvement

Figure 5.5. The process used to determine prognosis: step 3

The third step is the evaluation of the patient's response to treatment (figure 5.5). This step is fairly simple and considers how the patient may be evolving over time. The physician is asked to determine whether the patient's condition is getting worse, staying the same, or improving. Improvement means the patient reverses course and is clearly getting better. Stabilization implies the cessation of patient deterioration and evidence of signs of recovery. The response to treatment is not always linear in nature. Patient response to therapy might fluctuate due to factors that include lack of resolution of the initial insult, secondary effects or complications from treatment, or problems related to the hospital stay. It is frequently difficult to differentiate between these responses. In this third step, we will receive an answer to our question regarding which patients will survive after the initial insult.

Step 1. **BASELINE**
Chronological age
Previous level of function
Baseline organ damage

Step 2. **INITIAL ASSESSMENT**
Severity of the insult
New organ damage
Reversibility of the damage

Step 3. **RESPONSE TO TREATMENT**
Digression
Stabilization
Improvement

Step 4. **PROGNOSIS**
Death
Stabilization at a non-sustainable level
Recovery with further dysfunction
Complete recovery

Figure 5.6. The process used to determine prognosis: step 4

The fourth step is the determination of the patient's prognosis (figure 5.6). Prognosis includes two aspects: survival and function. Survival is of course easier to understand: *Is the patient going to live, or is he or she going to die?* Function is a more complex concept and refers to how effective one can expect the recovery to be. Function in this context refers to the ability of the patient to provide care for him- or herself. Sometimes patients can survive but will need help to function. The help required by each patient depends directly on his/her functional level, which is the term that has also been used to describe the patient's deficits and needs. The range of support needed by an individual patient can range from limited social support and supervision to personal help or personal care, or total care, and sometimes the need for permanent cardiovascular, respiratory, or nutritional support. An acceptable functional level is a term that has not been defined and is frequently a matter of debate, leading to disagreements between caregivers, patients, and families. The term "acceptable functional level" is difficult to define because, in addition to the complex medical factors, there are other equally complicated but important contributing factors, including social and religious beliefs, patients' and families' preferences, and available resources. For example, some patients and their families believe permanent ventilators, total peripheral nutrition, tube feedings, and/or cardiovascular support are unacceptable, while others believe that these support systems should be available on an ongoing basis.

All these issues come together in the final step. At this point, the physician will consider the patient's previous level of function, the severity of the insult, the possibility of further loss of function due to permanent organ damage, and the patient's response to treatment thus far, and decides whether the patient could recover (with or without additional impairment, is likely to stabilize at a sustainable or unsustainable level or is likely to die relatively quickly).

These determinations are not always easy to make. In medicine, there is frequently a "gray zone" when it comes to making these types of decisions. Improvement and stability do not necessarily imply the same outcome and should always be analyzed within the context of the projected patient function. For example, we can consider the case of a patient in a persistent vegetative state who begins breathing on his own; a patient admitted to the intensive care unit who is stable on permanent cardiovascular, pulmonary, and intravenous nutritional support; or a patient who is frail, demented, and frequently dehydrated due to poor self-care but will improve temporarily with intravenous hydration. While all three patients will improve temporarily in response to medical care, the long-term prognoses have not changed. Also the condition and prognosis of each patient may change (even slightly) as frequently as from one day to the next. The most straightforward scenario is the patient who has not stabilized and continues to deteriorate so that no one doubts that he or she is approaching death.

Unfortunately, sometimes the information needed to make a sound and careful judgment is not complete. At other times, the physician does not have the time to establish a fully empathetic relationship with the patient and his/her family. In many of these cases, the patient and family do not agree with the physician; fortunately sometimes the patient turns around and begins improving even before the physician has had the time to assess the situation in full.

The important point is that physicians need to have a structured format that they can use to analyze patient information and provide them with appropriate medical care. This is the only way physicians can regain control of health care processes, be consistent with the care provided, and navigate safely through the innumerable regulations and quality measures the system has imposed on them.

As we now have a clear understanding of the process used to determine patient prognosis, the next step will be to place these findings within the context of the regular practice of medicine.

CHAPTER 6

Prognosticating

In this final chapter, we summarize the information presented in the previous sections and highlight the benefits, limitations, and future promise of prognostication. Among our conclusions, we believe that physicians who are skilled in prognostication will be empowered to make the correct decisions for their patients and can protect them from unnecessary medications and therapies. Physicians who embrace this methodology will also be able to help their patients determine what their wishes might be during their final years of life.

Objectives

The goals of this section are as follows:

- To understand the benefits of prognostication
- To appreciate its limitations
- To understand how the system might improve the practice of medicine
- To learn how to identify and evaluate patients with potentially poor prognoses

Introduction

The practice of medicine has changed substantially during the past century. As a result, prognostication has taken on new meanings as the process has become increasingly more complex.

In earlier times, physicians clearly understood and appreciated the concept of death. There was nothing ambiguous about death. Once the heart stopped beating, the person in question was declared dead. However, with the development and availability of organ transplantation, the definition of death underwent a profound change. Now, death is defined by the absence of brain activity, which may disappear even when a patient has residual cardiac and respiratory function. Also, it was not long ago that a person who became disabled by trauma or disease and could not recover fast enough to "carry his/her own weight" was deemed unlikely to survive. Today, because we have the means to keep many of these patients alive with artificial support, humans gained some semblance of control over the processes leading to death.

With these new skills and the multiple variables that determine life expectancy, physicians find it difficult, if not impossible, to predict how much longer a patient is likely to live or when he or she is about to die. However, using the process of prognostication, a physician can determine what might be the best treatment in a given circumstance based on the characteristics and circumstances of the patient.

Benefits

The process of prognostication can help at all levels of care. At an office visit, the use of this process will permit the physician to recognize patient decline due to acute diseases or aging. Given this information, services such as physical therapy, home health, home-based meal delivery, and/or close supervision can be prescribed. Collectively, these services may prevent future problems and may even limit the rate of patient decline. Prognostication will also help the physician to avoid extensive testing as well as unnecessary and futile drugs, therapies, procedures, and screenings. The results of prognostication may also prompt the physician to engage in critical discussions regarding advance directives and offer the patient palliative care and/or hospice services when needed.

In the hospital, prognostication can help to shape the treatment offered to the patient and may prevent futile care. This process will assist staff in assessing end-of-life issues and may also help determine the most appropriate discharge plan. The role of the physician at the nursing home is similar and includes even more emphasis on quality of life and end-of-life issues.

Limitations

Patients who seem to be similar to one another and who are in similar situations may have completely different life spans because of different scientific and economic resources as well as the willingness to maintain life at all costs. These situations introduce a critical question of when a patient might be permitted to die. In other words, how can we differentiate between *prolonging the patient's life* versus *simply prolonging the process of dying*? Apart from the medical issues involved in this complex question, equally important are the associated moral issues, religious beliefs, societal values, quality of life, and economic factors. Most of all, it is critical to have a clear understanding of patient and family preferences for end-of-life care.

The physician responsible for the patient's care is tasked with providing his/her best judgment regarding the patient's prognosis. The physician must help to facilitate the resolution of all pertinent medical issues.

How to utilize the system

Prognostication is a structured method that can be used to process patient information. The goal of this process is to determine the possibility of patient survival and their likely level of function. Based on these estimates, the physician can then identify the best course of action. As we described in a previous chapter, the process includes four steps. As a first step, the physician can estimate the physiological reserve of a given patient. This information will dictate the aggressiveness of the treatment offered. Patients who are currently residing in nursing homes or dementia units, and/or carry a diagnosis of terminal disease, are likely to be candidates for less aggressive treatments that are oriented more toward palliative care and hospice. By contrast, patients with a high level of function and minimal organ damage might respond effectively to a curative approach with aggressive treatment. It is important to remember that age is the best predictor of low physiological reserve and shorter life expectancy in older healthy individuals.

The second step is the initial assessment. This will provide physicians with an opportunity to estimate the impact of the acute insult on the status of the patient. Patients who have been overwhelmed by the insult frequently die immediately or while undergoing assessment in the emergency department; patients who might (or might not) survive are frequently unstable and require treatment in the intensive care unit. More stable patients are typically managed by a routine medical ward. Prognostication might be applied to patients in the latter two groups. Subtracting the impact of new organ damage from the patient's baseline, together with a consideration of the natural history of the disease, will help the physician to determine what might be expected for each patient.

The third step focuses on the response of the patient to treatment. This information will provide insight into the likelihood of survival in some of the patients in the latter two groups. These are the patients that one needs to consider when contemplating questions about prolonging life or prolonging the process of dying. The likely outcome is more predictable for those patients who are likely to die if support systems (i.e., inotropics, pacemakers, and ventilators) are discontinued. The answer to this question may be somewhat different if the patient requires tube feeding and decubitus care, which can be provided at home or in a nursing home. However, these issues are frequently considered in dementia units, nursing homes, and sometimes at home when frail, and frequently demented patients are unable to eat or drink in amounts sufficient to sustain life.

The fourth step is the actual determination of the prognosis of the patient. There are three aspects to consider in this situation. The first aspect to consider is the possibility that the patient might survive, while the second refers to the treatment that most clearly benefits the patient, i.e., curative therapy *versus* palliative and/or hospice care. The final aspect considers the choice of the best level of care based on patient needs, remaining function, and resources. The act of working through the three different aspects of prognostication will provide the physician with a better perspective of a given patient's future and, indirectly, the risks, benefits, and consequences of current therapies and future recommendations.

While some patients die at home, at the site of an accident, or within the first few hours in the hospital, those who survive and require ongoing care can be classified into four groups based on their respective prognoses. The first group includes those patients who can be stabilized with high-level support, e.g., permanent mechanical ventilation or cardiovascular or nutritional support. These patients will require permanent skilled care either in a hospital or a specialized unit. These patients will die immediately if the support is discontinued. Those who are maintained in this state will return repeatedly to an acute care hospital for the treatment of complications and eventually become completely dependent before death. The second group, while similar in some ways to the first, includes patients requiring lower-level care (e.g., tracheotomy care, and/or tube feedings). These services can be provided in the home or at a nursing facility. However, these patients also return frequently to acute care facilities and most often also become completely dependent before death. The third group includes those patients who sustain some loss of function but can maintain life without extreme support. Depending on their previous level of function and the severity of the new deficits, these patients may also become dependent or partially dependent or may remain partially independent if provided with special equipment and/or environmental modifications. The fourth group includes patients who might eventually recover their baseline level of function and return to their previous living arrangements. However, it is critical to recognize that there may be overlap and unexpected changes. Many patient cases will fall between these strict definitions; others may move from one group to another over time.

However, by following the steps that outline the process of prognostication, a large number of patients will be classified appropriately. Again there will always be patients with unexpected outcomes. Likewise other patients and families may not agree to comply with the doctor's recommended plan despite the careful assessment of the patient's condition before prognostication.

It is important to remember that these decisions need to be discussed openly with caregivers, the family, and the patient. These individuals are responsible for the final decisions in all cases.

Identification and management of patients with poor prognoses

It is difficult to plan for the care of patients who do not stabilize or stabilize only when maintained on high-level support. These are the patients who are frequently evaluated by and receive treatment recommendations from different groups of task-oriented busy physicians who are concerned about meeting standards of care and productivity. The practice of medicine today is not focused on providing physicians with enough time to evaluate the benefits (or lack thereof) of the various treatment options for these patients.

Several tools are available that can be used to identify patients with a potentially poor prognosis. For example, the tool shown in figure 4.6 highlights frequent visits to the emergency department for the same problem, prolonged stays in the intensive care unit, or lack of response to treatment, as characteristics common to patients with a generally poor prognosis.

Another helpful tool that can be used at the bedside is shown in table 4.9. These are the criteria used by a hospice to determine patient eligibility for their services.

Physicians frequently persist with a curative approach for these patients because of the lack of clearly established alternative pathways. The next figure (figure 6.1) shows a pathway that might be used to proceed with these patients.

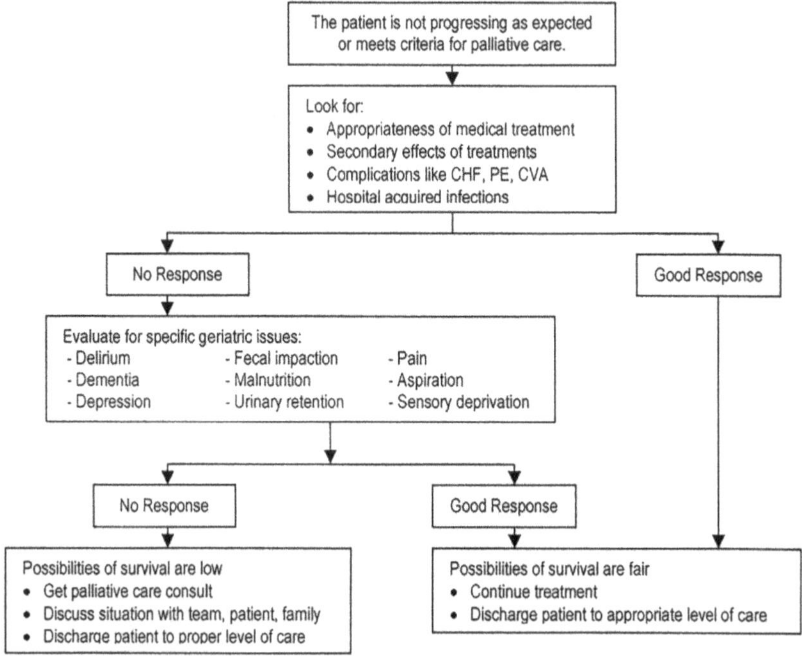

Figure 6.1. Flowchart used to manage patients in need of palliative care

The information shown in figure 6.1 addresses cases in which the patient's physiological strength is outweighed by the demands of the pathological process. As a group, these patients are more likely to succumb to secondary effects from medications and are more susceptible to hospital-acquired infections, aspiration pneumonia, malnutrition, muscle atrophy, delirium, and depression, among other complications. Of note, one might consider decreasing the demands on the failing physiological strength of the patient by identifying, avoiding, or treating these secondary problems to reverse the aforementioned imbalance.

Following this pathway does not guarantee that one will be "prolonging the patient's life" as opposed to "prolonging the process of dying." Nonetheless, the use of this process will provide physicians with some assurance that all significant aspects of the patient's care have been considered, even if the patient has not shown any signs of clinical improvement. This is important information, not only for the physician's peace of mind but also as a basis for communicating a poor prognosis to the patient and family and for discussing the options of curative treatments *versus* palliative care.

It is also critical to appreciate that an understanding of the diagnosis, prognosis, and treatment options is only the first step when one needs to explain the situation clearly and precisely to patients and their families. This is another very important and complex aspect of the practice of medicine that is beyond the scope of this book. The literature on palliative care and hospice is extensive and includes various approaches and ways of communicating these issues to patients and their families. Maintaining effective communication as part of the process of prognostication is certainly among the most intense and emotionally complex interactions a physician is likely to encounter in routine medical practice. Physicians must become proficient and comfortable with this interaction, even if they are unhappy with the prospect of delivering what is likely to be unhappy news.

The practice of medicine is currently at a crossroads. The knowledge acquired over the past several years, changes in expectations, overt industrialization, failure of the current economic system, and the scientific isolation in which medicine has developed have all led to the depersonalization of the practice of medicine. This has led to an unacceptable chasm separating the physician from the patient. The commonly held belief that appropriate medical care could keep everyone alive indefinitely ignores the fact that death is ultimately unavoidable once one reaches old age. As the population grows older, the needs of the average patient increase. The oldest patients are now weaker and present with numerous medical problems. Thus, given that progressive weakness is unavoidable and implicit in the process of aging, maintaining a strict focus on the disease process will not necessarily lead to clinical improvement in this patient population. Furthermore, all standards of care that lead to positive outcomes in younger and healthier patients might not be as effective for those who are older and frail.

Pressure from the medical industry, the public, and the system of care itself currently forces physicians to use the standards of care developed for a younger population to treat patients who are elderly and potentially frail. This creates a situation in which inappropriate and potentially unwanted and extremely expensive care, yet futile care, is administered to these patients.

Prognostication is a process that could help the physician to regain control of patient care. Using this process, physicians will be empowered to make the correct decisions regarding patient treatment and prevent the use of unnecessary medications and therapies. This will also provide them with the opportunity to educate their patients and help them to determine what their wishes might be during their final years of life.

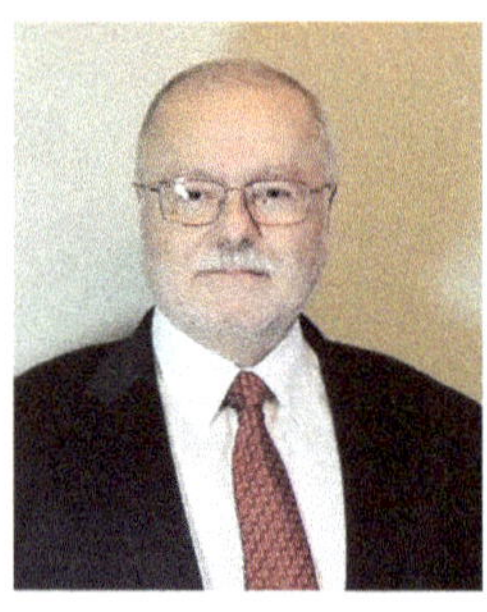

Bernardo Gutierrez is a retired medical doctor and assistant professor of medicine. Over his nearly fifty-year career in medicine, he practiced in cardiology for nearly ten years, starting with a residency at the Abood Shaio Hospital in Bogota, Colombia, after graduating at the top five of his class from Javeriana University in Bogota, Colombia, in 1972.

He immigrated to the United States in 1985, completing a residency in internal medicine at St. Luke's Hospital followed by a fellowship in geriatrics at Barnes-Jewish Hospital and St. Louis University Medical Center in St. Louis, Missouri, in 1991. Over the ensuing thirty years, Dr. Gutierrez practiced across the United States in varied settings including teaching hospitals, solo practice, veterans affairs, occupational medicine, emergency room, acute care, intensive care, skilled units, nursing homes, and terminal care. Over this time, he developed an interest and focus on the process of death. Dr. Gutierrez has made significant civic contributions, including two years of service to the Colombian National Social Health Service for poor rural health institutions and one year of medical service to the Veterans Affairs Medical Center in Oklahoma City, Oklahoma.

Dr. Gutierrez enjoys fishing, range shooting, traveling, and spending time with his family. He has been married for almost fifty years and has three adult children and five grandchildren. He and his wife are enjoying retirement between Central Florida and his hometown in Armenia, Colombia.